WORLD HEALTH ORGANIZATION

INTERNATIONAL AGENCY FOR RESEARCH ON CANCER

LABORATORY DECONTAMINATION AND DESTRUCTION OF CARCINOGENS IN LABORATORY WASTES: SOME ANTINEOPLASTIC AGENTS

EDITORS

M. CASTEGNARO, J. ADAMS, M.A. ARMOUR, J. BAREK,
J. BENVENUTO, C. CONFALONIERI, U. GOFF, S. LUDEMAN,
D. REED, E.B. SANSONE & G. TELLING

RC267
A1
I5
no.73
1985

IARC SCIENTIFIC PUBLICATIONS NO. 73

INTERNATIONAL AGENCY FOR RESEARCH ON CANCER
LYON
1985

Distributed for the International Agency for Research on Cancer by
Oxford University Press, Walton Street, Oxford OX2 6DP

London   New York   Toronto
Delhi   Bombay   Calcutta   Madras   Karachi
Kuala Lumpur   Singapore   Hong Kong   Tokyo
Nairobi   Dar es Salaam   Cape Town
Melbourne   Auckland

Oxford is a trade mark of Oxford University Press

Distributed in the United States
by Oxford University Press, New York

ISBN 92 832 1173 1
ISSN 0300-5085

© International Agency for Research on Cancer 1985
150 cours Albert Thomas, 69372 Lyon Cedex 08, France

PRINTED IN SWITZERLAND

The International Agency for Research on Cancer (IARC) was established in 1965 by the World Health Assembly, as an independently financed organization within the framework of the World Health Organization. The headquarters of the Agency are at Lyon, France.

The Agency conducts a programme of research concentrating particularly on the epidemiology of cancer and the study of potential carcinogens in the human environment. Its field studies are supplemented by biological and chemical research carried out in the Agency's laboratories in Lyon, and, through collaborative research agreements, in national research institutions in many countries. The Agency also conducts a programme for the education and training of personnel for cancer research.

The publications of the Agency are intended to contribute to the dissemination of authoritative information on different aspects of cancer research.

Publications in this series:

Aflatoxins B_1, B_2, G_1, G_2 (IARC Scientific Publications No. 37), 1980

Some N-Nitrosamines (IARC Scientific Publications No. 43), 1982

Some Polycyclic Aromatic Hydrocarbons (IARC Scientific Publications No. 49), 1983

Some Hydrazines (IARC Scientific Publications No. 54), 1983

Some N-Nitrosamides (IARC Scientific Publications No. 55), 1983

Some Haloethers (IARC Scientific Publications No. 61), 1984

Some Aromatic Amines and 4-Nitrobiphenyl (IARC Scientific Publications No. 64), 1985

CONTENTS

FOREWORD

While previous monographs in the series *Laboratory Decontamination and Destruction of Carcinogens in Laboratory Wastes* have been of interest mainly to workers with laboratory facilities, this volume, dealing with antineoplastic agents, addresses not only those persons but also and even more so hospital and pharmacy staff who are currently exposed to these substances. This volume has, therefore, been prepared and edited with special attention to the latter groups of persons, and it is hoped that it will contribute to increasing safety in hospitals, as well as in laboratories where the synthesis, testing and analysis of antineoplastic agents is carried out.

The IARC wishes to acknowledge the support of the Division of Safety of the National Institutes of Health, USA, towards the preparation of this volume and also wishes to thank all the scientists who took part in the validation of the methods presented in this document and in their development.

L. TOMATIS, M.D.
Director, IARC

PREAMBLE

Biomedical research involving toxic chemicals, including carcinogens, inevitably results in the production of waste products containing these potentially hazardous materials. The safe and environmentally sound disposal of these wastes has become an ever-increasing concern of the governments, research institutions, investigators and private citizens, and has resulted in a significant number of enquiries for recommended disposal methods. During our investigation of this area, two significant problems became apparent: (1) there is a paucity of published information on the destruction and disposal of carcinogenic wastes, and (2), of the published methods available, few have been thoroughly evaluated or rigorously tested to ensure that the destruction of the parent compound is complete and that the reaction by-products are relatively innocuous.

In September 1978, The Division of Safety, National Institutes of Health, USA, established with the International Agency for Research on Cancer a special programme to develop an authoritive series of monographs on methods for the destruction and disposal of carcinogenic waste from biomedical research laboratories. We wanted to draw upon the experience of the Agency in bringing together internationally recognized scientific experts to review critically data applicable to the destruction and disposal of carcinogenic waste, to recommend destruction strategies, to develop new methods where necessary, and to subject the designated methods to interlaboratory collaborative verification to confirm their efficacy. The current volume is the eighth of a series that has thus far included disposal methods for aflatoxins, N-nitrosamines, polycyclic aromatic hydrocarbons, hydrazines, N-nitrosamides, haloethers and aromatic amines.

This volume focuses on methods for the safe destruction of a chemically diverse group of antineoplastic chemotherapeutic drugs. Interest in such methods has increased with the recognition that these very effective chemotherapeutic agents may place health workers at risk if they are inadvertently exposed to the drug during its preparation or administration to patients. This volume is intended to supplement earlier guidance from the National Institutes of Health for the safe handling of parenteral antineoplastic drugs, by providing safe and effective methods to destroy these materials chemically prior to disposal. The methods described herein are intended for use not only in laboratories but also in hospitals, clinics and pharmacies where other options for the safe disposal of these drugs may be limited.

Throughout the period of this programme, the Agency and the Division of Safety have encouraged individual scientists and laboratories in the international community to contribute to the development of methods and to participate in validation studies. It is our hope that this programme serves as a catalyst for stimulating research in this area and for sharing the results of such investigations.

W. Emmett Barkley, PhD
Director,
Division of Safety,
National Institutes of Health, USA

ANTINEOPLASTIC AGENTS CONSIDERED

The following antineoplastic agents were considered in this volume. The methods described for the destruction of specific compounds or groups may be applicable to other compounds from the same group; however, when dealing with other compounds, the efficiency of the methods should first be verified.

Antineoplastic agent	Chemical Abstracts Services Registry Number
Doxorubicin	23214-92-8
Daunorubicin	20830-81-3
Methotrexate	59-05-2
Dichloromethotrexate	528-74-5
Cyclophosphamide	6055-19-2
Ifosfamide	3778-73-2
Vincristine sulfate	2068-78-2
Vinblastine sulfate	143-67-9
6-Thioguanine	154-42-7
6-Mercaptopurine	50-42-2
Cisplatin	15663-27-1
Streptozotocin	18883-66-4
Chlorozotocin	54749-90-5
Lomustine	13010-47-4
Carmustine*	154-93-8
Semustine*	13909-09-6
Urea, N-(2-chloroethyl)-N'-(2,6-dioxo-3-piperidinyl)-N-nitroso- (PCNU)*	13909-02-9
Melphalan*	148-82-3

* For these compounds, no method can be recommended at this time.

INTRODUCTION

Carcinogenicity

The carcinogenic activity of a number of antineoplastic agents has been studied extensively in several animal species. For 13 of the 18 compounds listed above, the data on carcinogenicity have been evaluated by working groups of experts (International Agency for Research on Cancer, 1974, 1975, 1976, 1978, 1981) and the compounds classified into one of the three following groups (International Agency for Research on Cancer, 1982; Table 1):

Group 1: Carcinogenic to humans

Group 2: Probably carcinogenic to humans. This category includes exposures for which, at one extreme, the evidence of human carcinogenicity is almost sufficient, as well as exposures for which, at the other extreme, it is inadequate. To reflect this range, the category was divided into higher (Group A) and lower (Group B) degrees of evidence.

Group 3: Cannot be classified as to its carcinogenicity to humans.

The other five compounds have not been evaluated for carcinogenicity by IARC working groups. However, semustine and chlorozotocin have been reported to be carcinogenic to rats (Habs *et al.*, 1979; Eisenbrand & Habs, 1980; Eisenbrand *et al.*, 1981). No data were found in the literature concerning the carcinogenicity of PCNU, 6-thioguanine and dichloromethotrexate. In view of the carcinogenic activity of other nitrosourea drugs, PCNU should, for practical purposes, be considered to be carcinogenic.

Analytical methods

Doxorubicin and daunorubicin

Early attempts to analyse doxorubicin and daunorubicin made use of paper and thin-layer chromatography (TLC) coupled with ultraviolet (UV) detection (Arcamone *et al.*, 1969). The fluorescent characteristics of these two compounds have also been used to establish fluorimetric assay methods for their determination in biological fluids and tissues (Finkel *et al.*, 1969; Dusonchet *et al.*, 1971; Schwartz, 1973); however, these methods have some disadvantages due to lack of specificity. The use of high-performance liquid chromatography (HPLC), coupled to electrochemical, fluorimetric or UV detection systems, has greatly improved the specificity of the analytical methods (Eksborg, 1978; Pierce & Jatlow, 1979; Andrews *et al.*, 1980; Robert, 1980; Sepaniak & Yeung, 1980; Brown *et al.*, 1981; Haneke *et al.*, 1981; Shinozawa & Oda, 1981; White & Zarembo, 1981; Akpofure *et al.*, 1982; Bolanowska *et al.*, 1983; Bots *et al.*, 1983) as well as their sensitivity.

Other methods, including isotachophoretic determination (Akedo & Shinkai, 1982), gas chromatography (GC)/mass spectrometry (MS) of trimethylsilylated de-

Table 1. Classification of antineoplastic agents on the basis of degree of evidence for carcinogenicity [a]

Agent	Classification
Doxorubicin	2B
Daunorubicin	No data on humans; carcinogenic to rats and mice
Methotrexate	3
Cyclophosphamide	1
Ifosfamide	No data on humans; limited evidence of carcinogenicity to rats and mice
Vincristine sulfate	3
Vinblastine sulfate	3
6-Mercaptopurine	3
Cisplatin	2B
Streptozotocin	No data on humans; carcinogenic to rats, mice and hamsters
Lomustine	2B
Carmustine	2B
Melphalan	1

[a] From International Agency for Research on Cancer (1982)

rivatives (Andrews *et al.*, 1982a) have been used to determine doxorubicin and daunorubicin and their metabolites in biological fluids. Radioimmunoassay techniques for the determination of doxorubicin in plasma have been evaluated by Piall *et al.* (1982). Methods of analysis of doxorubicin have been reviewed (Vigevani & Williamson, 1980).

Methotrexate and dichloromethotrexate

Several methods that have been used for the analysis of methotrexate have been reviewed by Chamberlin *et al.* (1976), including biological assays, polarographic assays, spectrophotometric methods and chromatographic techniques (paper chromatography, column chromatography and TLC). However, at the present time, HPLC is the most widely used technique for the analysis of methotrexate. It may be coupled either with a UV detection system (Chatterji & Gallelli, 1977; Benvenuto *et al.*, 1981; Chen & Chiou, 1981; Breithaupt *et al.*, 1982; Cairnes & Evans, 1982; Battelli *et al.*, 1983; Feyns *et al.*, 1982), with a coulometric detection system (Dutrieu & Delmotte, 1983) or with field desorption mass spectrometry (Przybylski *et al.*, 1982).

This method has also recently been used for the analysis of dichloromethotrexate (Keller & Ensminger, 1982), using a UV detection system.

Other methods, such as spectrophotometry, colorimetry and differential pulse polarography (Ellaithy et al., 1982), or enzymatic assay (Scheufler, 1981; Akira et al., 1982), have also recently been used for the determination of methotrexate.

Cyclophosphamide and ifosfamide

Methods of analysis for cyclophosphamide and ifosfamide generally involve their extraction in an organic solvent, followed either by direct GC separation coupled with MS, nitrogen/phosphorous or electron capture detection systems (Boughton et al., 1972; Jackson & Reynolds, 1972; Whiting et al., 1978; Benvenuto et al., 1981; Daldrup et al., 1981; Van den Bosch et al., 1981; De Bruin et al., 1983) or with GC analysis after derivatization with hexafluorobutyric anhydride (Holdiness & Morgan, 1983) or trifluoracetic anhydride (Pantarotto et al., 1974; Whiting et al., 1978).

Other chromatographic techniques have been used, including TLC (Völker et al., 1974; Gattavecchia et al., 1983) and HPLC using photoconductivity detection (McKinley, 1981) or UV detection (Kensler et al., 1979).

Spectrophotometric microdetermination of phosphorus has also been used to determine cyclophosphomide (Hassan & Eldesouki, 1981).

Vincristine and vinblastine sulfates

Methods for the analysis of vincristine and vinblastine sulfate were reviewed by Burns (1972) and include colorimetric assays, direct spectrophotometry and TLC; the latter method can separate the two compounds (Cone et al., 1963). More recently, TLC has been proposed for use in identifying the metabolic products of vincristine sulfate and to determine vincristine in biological samples after extraction into benzene (El Dareer, 1977). TLC has also been used to classify vinblastine among other compounds exhibiting anti-tumour properties (Issaq et al., 1977). TLC separation of vincristine from vinblastine sulfate and other impurities, followed by densitometric analysis, has been used by Panas et al. (1979) to determine the purity of vincristine sulfate.

HPLC has also been proposed for analysing vincristine and vinblastine sulfates separately (Görög et al., 1977; Benvenuto et al., 1981; Keller & Ensminger, 1982). A method using titrimetric determination of sulfate ions has been proposed for analysing solutions of vincristine or vinblastine sulfate (Hoor & Toth, 1981), but this method lacks specificity. Room temperature phosphorescence can also be used to analyse vinblastine sulfate (Bower & Winefordner, 1978); and differential pulse polarography has also been used for the determination of vinblastine (Rusling et al., 1984).

6-Thioguanine and 6-mercaptopurine

Methods for the analysis of 6-mercaptopurine have been reviewed (Benezra & Foss, 1978) and include spectrophotometry, polarography (Smith & Elving, 1962;

Dryhurst, 1969) and chromatographic techniques (TLC, GC, HPLC). TLC and GC conditions for the analysis of 6-mercaptopurine are also given by Daldrup *et al.* (1981).

At present, HPLC coupled with UV detection seems to be the method of choice for the direct analysis of either 6-mercaptopurine (Fell *et al.*, 1979; De Abreu *et al.*, 1982; Narang *et al.*, 1982; Tsutsumi *et al.*, 1982) or 6-thioguanine (Breithaupt & Goebel, 1981; Andrews *et al.*, 1982b).

6-Mercaptopurine has also been analysed by HPLC/spectrofluorimetry of its 6-sulfonate derivative, obtained by oxidation with acid chromate (Hirose & Tawa, 1983). Spectrofluorimetric detection of the sulfonate derivative has also been used after HPLC separation of 6-mercaptopuridine and on-line derivatization with chromate (Jonkers *et al.*, 1982).

Cisplatin

Flameless absorption spectrophotometry has been proposed for the analysis of platinum in biological samples (Priesner *et al.*, 1981; Cano *et al.*, 1982); however, this method allows analysis only of total platinum and does not differentiate between platinum-containing compounds. The use of differential pulse polarography after pretreatment of the sample is more specific (Bartošek *et al.*, 1982, 1983; Brabec *et al.*, 1983; Vrána *et al.*, 1983).

Use of HPLC significantly improves the specificity of methods for the analysis of cisplatin. It has been used coupled with UV detection for direct determination (Hincal *et al.*, 1979; Mariani *et al.*, 1980) or for analysis after derivatization with diethyldithiocarbanate (Bannister *et al.*, 1979); HPLC may also be coupled with electrochemical detection (Bannister *et al.*, 1983; Krull *et al.*, 1983) or with UV and off-line atomic absorption spectrophotometry (Chang *et al.*, 1978).

A number of HPLC systems that can be used for the analysis of cisplatin have been tested by Riley *et al.* (1981, 1982, 1983). A solvent-generated ion-exchange system seems the method of choice for the chromatographic separation of various platinum complexes.

Nitrosourea drugs

Slightly modified versions of the early method for the analysis of carmustine, with Bratton-Marschall reagent (Loo & Dion, 1965), are still used (Colvin *et al.*, 1980; Vachek *et al.*, 1982).

Other means of analysing for these compounds include differential pulse polarography (Bartošek *et al.*, 1978; Vachek *et al.*, 1982) and various chromatographic techniques. TLC analysis of streptozotocin has been discussed by Rudas (1972), but most developments have been in the use of GC and HPLC. Semustine has been analysed by GC after derivatization to the semicarbazide by sodium tetrahydroborate (III) (Caddy & Idowu, 1982a) or formation of its trifluoroacetyl derivative (Caddy & Idowu, 1982b). Smith *et al.* (1981) and Smith and Cheung (1982) also used derivatization with trifluoroacetic acid anhydride followed by GC/MS to analyse semustine, lomustine and carmustine. Formation of an *O*-methyl carbamate derivative followed by GC/nitrogen-specific detection analysis or GC/MS has been proposed by Weinkam and Liu (1982); and direct chemical ionization MS has been used by Weinkam *et al.* (1978). HPLC techniques appear to have received less attention than GC; they have been used, coupled with UV detection, for studies of the stability of carmustine, lomustine and semustine (May *et al.*, 1975; Reed *et al.*, 1975; Krull *et al.*, 1981; Aukerman *et al.*, 1983).

Melphalan

Little information has been published concerning the analysis of melphalan, but it appears that chromatographic techniques are the methods of choice. HPLC has been used, coupled with either a UV detection system (Flora *et al.*, 1979; Bosanquet & Gilby, 1982) or with spectrofluorimetry (Egan *et al.*, 1981; Woodhouse & Henderson, 1982).

After treatment with trifluoracetic acid and diazomethane, melphalan can be analysed as the *N*-trifluoracetyl methylester derivative by GC/MS (Pallante *et al.*, 1980).

RECOMMENDED METHODS OF DEGRADATION

INTRODUCTION

Previous monographs in this series have been of interest mainly to workers in specialized analytical facilities, whereas the present monograph covers a group of compounds widely used in hospital clinics and pharmacies. In such areas, it is less likely that fume cupboards and other facilities and equipment for handling toxic hazardous chemicals are available; hence, methods for the destruction of antineoplastic agents have been developed with the needs of medical staff in mind.

In the description of each method, a number of potential hazards have been identified. However, it must be recognized that no attempt has been made to provide comprehensive guidelines for safe working conditions and that adherence to a code of good practice is essential.

Eight destruction methods have been tested for use on one or more of the listed antineoplastic agents. The efficiency of destruction achieved with the various methods was evaluated by collaborative study, and the residues produced were tested for mutagenicity using the Ames *Salmonella* mutation assay (Ames *et al.*, 1975; Bartsch *et al.*, 1980). Several strains – TA1530, TA1535, TA98, TA100, TA102 or UTH8414 – were used to test the residues of each destruction method. If not mentioned, no mutagenic residue was detected; however, it should be recognized that absence of mutagenic activity in residual solutions does not necessarily imply lack of toxicity or of other adverse biological or environmental effects. It should be noted that a change in the matrix of a pharmaceutical preparation may lead to significant changes in the efficiency of a destruction method. In such cases, therefore, the efficiency of the method should be verified.

Fifteen methods were tested for the destruction of the eighteen antineoplastic agents.

Doxorubicin and daunorubicin

Two methods were evaluated:

(1) Oxidation with potassium permanganate (0.3 mol/L) in sulfuric acid (3 mol/L) solution. This method gave acceptable results, except for doxorubicin, for which a mutagenic effect was detectable with *Salmonella typhimurium* strain TA102.
(2) Oxidation with 5 or 10% sodium hypochlorite solution. This method resulted in acceptable chemical degradation but was rejected due to mutagenic activity of the residues.

Methotrexate and dichloromethotrexate

Three methods were evaluated:

(1) Oxidation with potassium permanganate (0.3 mol/L) in sulfuric acid (3 mol/L) solution; tested on both methotrexate and dichloromethotrexate
(2) Oxidation with aqueous alkaline potassium permanganate; tested only on methotrexate

(3) Oxidation with a 30-fold excess of sodium hypochlorite solution; tested only on methotrexate

All three methods gave acceptable results.

Cyclophosphamide and ifosfamide

Three methods were evaluated:

(1) Alkaline hydrolysis in the presence of dimethylformamide. This method gave acceptable results for both compounds.
(2) Acid hydrolysis followed by addition of sodium thiosulfate and alkaline hydrolysis. This method gave acceptable results only for cyclophosphamide. Residues from the destruction of ifosfamide showed mutagenic activity, and the method was rejected for use with this compound.
(3) Oxidation with potassium permanganate (0.2 mol/L) in sulfuric acid (0.5 mol/L) solution. This method resulted in acceptable chemical destruction of both compounds but was rejected because of high mutagenic activity in the residues.

Vincristine sulfate and vinblastine sulfate

The only method tested, oxidation with potassium permanganate (0.3 mol/L) in sulfuric acid (3 mol/L) solution, gave acceptable results.

6-Thioguanine and 6-mercaptopurine

The only method tested, oxidation with potassium permanganate (0.04 mol/L) in sulfuric acid (3 mol/L) solution, gave acceptable results.

Cisplatin

Three methods were evaluated:

(1) Reduction with zinc powder. This method gave acceptable results.
(2) Reaction with sodium diethyldithiocarbamate. No analytical method was found suitable to verify the level of destruction; however, no mutagenic activity was detected in the residues and the method was accepted on this basis.
(3) Oxidation with potassium permanganate (0.02, 0.1 and 0.3 mol/L) in sulfuric acid solution (3 mol/L). No analytical method was found suitable to verify the level of destruction; however, since the residues showed high mutagenic activity, the method was rejected.

N-Nitrosourea drugs

(1) Cleavage with hydrogen bromide in glacial acetic acid. The method gave acceptable results for lomustine, chlorozotocin and streptozotocin. Destruction of PCNU was not reproducible, and residues from carmustine and semustine showed mutagenic activity.
(2) Oxidation with a saturated solution of potassium permanganate in 3 mol/L sulfuric acid solution of either the pure compound or of solutions containing di-

methylformamide (DMF) or dimethylsulfoxide (DMSO). The method was satisfactory only for streptozotocin. For lomustine, carmustine, semustine, PCNU and chlorozotocin, chemical destruction of the drugs was satisfactory but the method was rejected on the basis of the mutagenic activity of the residues.

It should be noted that a method for the treatment of aqueous spills has been validated only for streptozotocin.

Melphalan

The only method tested, oxidation with potassium permanganate (0.3 mol/L) in sulfuric acid (3 mol/L) solution, gave satisfactory chemical destruction but was rejected because of high mutagenic activity in the residues.

It is important to note that methods that work successfully for the destruction of some compounds may not work on other compounds of the same class or on other classes of compounds.

For example, oxidation with potassium permanganate/sulfuric acid solution has been used successfully for the destruction of several classes of compounds (Castegnaro *et al.*, 1980, 1982, 1983a,b,c, 1985). This method gave satisfactory results with some of the antineoplastic agents studied (see above), but failed with others, such as the majority of the *N*-nitrosourea drugs. Similarly, denitrosation with hydrogen bromide in glacial acetic acid worked for *N*-nitrosamines and *N*-nitrosamides (Castegnaro *et al.*, 1982, 1983c), but for only three of the six *N*-nitrosoureas tested. Sodium hypochlorite, often recommended for general destruction, could not be used for doxorubicin, daunorubicin, *N*-nitrosamines or polycyclic aromatic hydrocarbons, but could be used for aflatoxins (Castegnaro *et al.*, 1980) and hydrazines (Castegnaro *et al.*, 1983b).

When dealing with quantities larger than those described in the methods, it should be borne in mind that even efficiencies of destruction in excess of 99.5% can result in the presence of significant quantities of antineoplastic agents in the residues.

Incineration of wastes containing antineoplastic agents is widely practised. Unfortunately, it has not yet proved possible to develop a validated method. On the one hand, the conditions of incineration vary widely between different installations; on the other hand, the technical difficulties of testing flue gases for the possible presence of volatile carcinogens are considerable.

The final test of the methods described in the following sections benefited from revision by the group that took part in the validation studies.

COLLABORATING ORGANIZATIONS

Collaborative studies of the methods described in this document were carried out with representatives from the following organizations:

Department of Chemistry, The University of Alberta, Edmonton, Alberta T6G 2G2, Canada

Department of Analytical Chemistry, Charles University, Albertov 2030, 128 40 Prague 2, Czechoslovakia

Department of Pharmacy and Chemotherapy Research, University of Texas System Cancer Center, M.D. Anderson Hospital & Tumor Institute, 6723 Bertner Avenue, Houston, TX 77030, USA

Pharmaceutical Research & Development, Farmitalia Carlo Erba, Via Carlo Imbonati 24, 20159 Milan, Italy

New England Institute for Life Sciences, 125 Second Avenue, Waltham, MA 02154, USA

Department of Chemistry, The Catholic University of America, Washington DC 20064, USA

Oregon State University, Department of Biochemistry and Biophysics, Cornwallis, OR 97331, USA

Environmental Control & Research Program, NCI-Frederick Cancer Research Facility, PO Box B, Frederick, MD 21701, USA

Unilever Research, Colworth Laboratory, Sharnbrook, Beds MK44 1LQ, UK

Unit of Environmental Carcinogens and Host Factors, Division of Environmental Carcinogenesis, International Agency for Research on Cancer, 150 Cours Albert Thomas, 69372 Lyon Cedex 08, France

METHODS INDEX:

1. METHODS RECOMMENDED FOR SPECIFIC WASTE CATEGORIES CONTAINING METHOTREXATE OR DICHLOROMETHOTREXATE

Waste category	Recommended destruction method no. (in order of preference)	
	Methotrexate	Dichloromethotrexate
Solid compounds	3, 4, 2	2
Aqueous solutions and pharmaceutical solutions	3, 4, 2	2
Solutions in volatile organic solvents	3, 4, 2	2
Solutions in DMF and DMSO	2	2
Glassware	3, 4, 2	2
Spills of solid compounds	4, 3, 2	2
Spills of aqueous solutions and pharmaceutical solutions	4, 3, 2	2
Spills of solutions in volatile organic solvents	4, 3, 2	2

2. METHODS RECOMMENDED FOR SPECIFIC WASTE CATEGORIES CONTAINING CYCLOPHOSPHAMIDE OR IFOSFAMIDE

Waste category	Recommended destruction method no.	
	Cyclophosphamide	Ifosfamide
Solid compounds	5 or 6	5
Aqueous solutions and pharmaceutical preparations	5 or 6	5
Solutions in DMF	5 or 6	5
Solutions in volatile organic solvents	5 or 6	5
Solutions in DMSO	5 or 6	5
Glassware	5 or 6	5
Spills of solid compounds	5 or 6	5
Spills of aqueous solutions or of solutions in DMF or DMSO	5 or 6	5
Spills of solutions in volatile organic solvents	5 or 6	5

3. METHODS RECOMMENDED FOR SPECIFIC WASTE CATEGORIES CONTAINING CISPLATIN

Waste category	Recommended destruction method no. (in order of preference)
Solid compound	10, 9
Aqueous solutions and pharmaceutical solutions	10, 9
Solutions in water – miscible solvents	9
Glassware	10, 9
Spills	10

4. METHODS RECOMMENDED FOR SPECIFIC WASTE CATEGORIES CONTAINING CHLOROZOTOCIN, STREPTOZOTOCIN OR LOMUSTINE

Waste category	Recommended destruction method no. (in order of preference)		
	Chlorozotocin	Streptozotocin	Lomustine
Solid compounds	11	11, 12	11
Pharmaceutical preparations (solids)	11	11, 12	11
Aqueous solutions		12	11
Pharmaceutical solutions		12	
Solutions in volatile organic solvents	11	11, 12	11
Solutions in DMF or DMSO		12	
Solutions in ethanol or methanol	11	12, 11	11
Glassware	11	11, 12	11
Spills of solid compounds	11	11, 12	11
Spills of liquid or pharmaceutical preparations		12	
Spills of solutions in volatile organic solvents	11	11, 12	11

METHODS

METHOD 1: DESTRUCTION OF DOXORUBICIN AND DAUNORUBICIN USING POTASSIUM PERMANGANATE/SULFURIC ACID

1. SCOPE AND FIELD OF APPLICATION

This method specifies a procedure for the destruction of doxorubicin and daunorubicin in the following wastes: solid compounds (6.1), aqueous solutions (6.2), pharmaceutical preparations (6.3), solutions in volatile organic solvents (6.4), solutions in dimethylsulfoxide (DMSO) (6.5), glassware (6.6), spills of solid compounds (6.7), spills of aqueous solutions or of pharmaceutical preparations (6.8) and spills of solutions in volatile organic solvents (6.9).

The method has been tested collaboratively using 10 mg doxorubicin (pharmaceutical preparation) and a solution containing 50 mg daunorubicin in 3 mL DMSO. The method affords better than 99% degradation for the samples tested.

The residues produced by this method were tested for mutagenicity using *Salmonella typhimurium* strains TA98, TA100 and TA102 with and without metabolic activation. No mutagenic activity was detected with residues from daunorubicin, but twice the background level of spontaneous mutants was seen with the highest concentration of residues from doxorubicin in *Salmonella typhimurium* strain TA102.

2. PRINCIPLE

Destruction is effected by oxidation with a solution of potassium permanganate in sulfuric acid.

3. HAZARDS

3.1 *From doxorubicin and daunorubicin*

Doxorubicin and daunorubicin are potentially carcinogenic to humans, have high systemic toxicity and are corrosive on skin contact. Exposure to these compounds should be avoided.

A number of guidelines for the safe handling of antineoplastic agents have been published (Knowles & Virden, 1980; Davis, 1981; Harrison, 1981; Zimmerman *et al.*, 1981; Anderson *et al.*, 1982; National Institutes of Health, 1982; Jones *et al.*, 1983; Solimando, 1983; Stolar *et al.*, 1983; National Study Commission on Cytotoxic Exposure, 1984; American Society of Hospital Pharmacists, 1985).

3.2 *Other hazards*

Concentrated sulfuric acid and sodium hydroxide are corrosive and should be handled with care.

Care should be taken in the preparation of solutions of potassium permanganate in sulfuric acid; never add solid potassium permanganate to concentrated sulfuric acid.

The dilution of concentrated sulfuric acid with water is an extremely exothermic reaction; always add the acid to the water, never the reverse, and remove heat by cooling in a cold-water bath.

Potassium permanganate is a strong oxidizing agent; care must be taken not to mix it with concentrated reducing agents.

In case of skin contact with corrosive chemicals, wash the skin with flowing water for at least 15 min.

4. REAGENTS

4.1 *For destruction*

Potassium permanganate	Technical grade
Sulfuric acid (concentrated)	Specific gravity, 1.84 (about 18 mol/L); technical grade
Sulfuric acid solution	3 mol/L, aqueous (see Hazards, 3.2)
Potassium permanganate/sulfuric acid solution	To 100 mL of 3 mol/L sulfuric acid solution, add 4.7 g solid potassium permanganate.

NOTE: The reagent should always be freshly prepared on the day of use.

Ascorbic acid or sodium bisulfite	Technical grade
Ascorbic acid or sodium bisulfite solution	$\simeq$ 50 g/L, aqueous
Sodium hydroxide	Technical grade
Sodium hydroxide solution	$\simeq$ 2 mol/L, aqueous (8 g/100 mL)
Sodium carbonate	Technical grade

4.2 *For analysis*

Ascorbic acid	Analytical grade
Water	Redistilled from glass

Acetonitrile	HPLC grade
Phosphoric acid	Analytical grade; specific gravity, 1.71
Potassium dihydrogenphosphate	Analytical grade

5. APPARATUS

Usual laboratory equipment and the following item: liquid chromatograph equipped with a spectrofluorimetric detection system, capable of determining 0.2 ng/mL of drug under the following conditions: excitation, 470 nm; emission, 565 nm.

6. PROCEDURE

Thirty mg of doxorubicin or daunorubicin dissolved in 10 mL of 3 mol/L sulfuric acid are destroyed by 1 g potassium permanganate in 2 h.

6.1 *Solid compounds*

6.1.1   Dissolve in 3 mol/L sulfuric acid to obtain a maximum content of 3 mg/mL.

6.1.2   Place flask on a magnetic stirrer; add about 1 g potassium permanganate per 10 mL of solution from 6.1.1.

6.1.3   Allow to react 2 h with stirring,

6.1.4   If desired, check for completeness of degradation using the procedure described in Section 7.

6.1.5   Neutralize with 8 g/100 mL sodium hydroxide solution, and discard.

6.2 *Aqueous solutions*

6.2.1   If necessary, dilute with water to obtain a maximum concentration of 3 mg/mL.

6.2.2   Add slowly, with stirring, enough concentrated sulfuric acid to obtain a 3 mol/L solution and allow to cool to room temperature (see 3.2., Hazards).

6.2.3   Proceed as in 6.1.2 to 6.1.5.

6.3 *Pharmaceutical preparations*

NOTE: To avoid frothing, add potassium permanganate in small increments.

6.3.1   Liquids: proceed as in 6.2, using twice the amount of potassium permanganate.

6.3.2   Solids: dissolve in water and treat as in 6.2, using twice the amount of potassium permanganate.

6.4 *Solutions in volatile organic solvents*

6.4.1   Remove solvent by evaporation, using a rotary evaporator under reduced pressure.

6.4.2   Proceed as in 6.1.1 to 6.1.5.

6.5 *Solutions in DMSO*

6.5.1   Dilute with water to not more than 20% DMSO and to not more than 3 mg/mL of drug.

6.5.2   Proceed as in 6.2, using twice the amount of potassium permanganate.

6.6 *Glassware*

6.6.1   Immerse in a freshly prepared solution of potassium permanganate/sulfuric acid. Allow to react 2 h.

6.6.2   Clean the glass by immersion in a solution of ascorbic acid or sodium bisulfite.

6.7 *Spills of solid compounds*

6.7.1   Isolate the area, and put on suitable protective clothing.

6.7.2   Pour an excess of potassium permanganate/sulfuric acid solution over the contaminated area. If the purple colour fades, add more potassium permanganate. Allow to react 2 h.

6.7.3   Decolourize the surface with a solution of ascorbic acid or sodium bisulfite.

6.7.4   Neutralize by addition of solid sodium carbonate.

6.7.5   Remove the decontamination mixture with an absorbent material.

6.7.6   Discard.

6.7.7   If desired, check the surface for completeness of removal by wiping it with methanol and analysing the wipe (see Section 7).

6.8 *Spills of aqueous solutions or of pharmaceutical preparations*

    6.8.1   Proceed as in 6.7.

6.9 *Spills of solutions in volatile organic solvents*

    6.9.1   Isolate the area, and put on suitable protective clothing.

    6.9.2   Allow the solvent to evaporate.

    6.9.3   Proceed as in 6.7.2 to 6.7.7.

7. ANALYSIS FOR COMPLETENESS OF DEGRADATION

7.1 Add ascorbic acid until the solution becomes colourless.

7.2 Analyse by HPLC, using the following conditions, or any other suitable HPLC reverse-phase chromatography system:

Column: 25 cm × 3.6 mm i.d., Partisil ODS-2 10 μm

Precolumn: 6.5 cm × 3.6 mm i.d., filled with CO:Pell ODS 30–38 μm

Eluant: Isocratic system. Acetonitrile:0.01 mol/L potassium dihydrogenphosphate in 0.02 mol/L phosphoric acid (45:55)

Flow rate: 1.5 mL/min

Injection volume: 50 μL

Spectrofluorimetric analysis: excitation, 470 nm; emission, 565 nm

NOTE: The high sensitivity required for the fluorescence detection system is necessary because of the high mutagenic activity of the compound. If such a detector is not available, it may be possible to achieve the required limit of detection by the use of extraction/concentration techniques (Andrews *et al.*, 1980), or by slightly changing the eluant and the flow rate to permit the use of 500-μL injections.

8. SCHEMATIC REPRESENTATION OF PROCEDURE

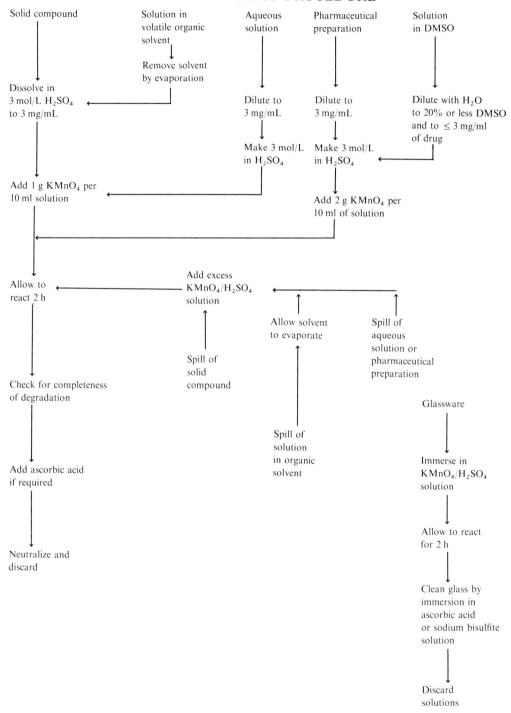

9.   ORIGIN OF METHOD

Castegnaro, M., Brouet, I. & Michelon, J.
International Agency for Research on Cancer
150 Cours Albert Thomas
69372 Lyon Cedex 08, France

Contact point: M. CASTEGNARO

METHOD 2: DESTRUCTION OF METHOTREXATE AND DICHLOROMETHOTREXATE USING POTASSIUM PERMANGANATE/SULFURIC ACID

1. SCOPE AND FIELD OF APPLICATION

This method specifies a procedure for the destruction of methotrexate and dichloromethotrexate in the following wastes: solid compounds (6.1), aqueous solutions (6.2), injectable pharmaceutical preparations (6.3), solutions in volatile organic solvents (6.4), solutions in dimethylsulfoxide (DMSO) or dimethylformamide (DMF) (6.5), glassware (6.6), spills of solid compounds (6.7), spills of aqueous solutions or of injectable pharmaceutical preparations (6.8) and spills of solutions in volatile organic solvents (6.9).

The method has been tested collaboratively using 5 mg methotrexate (pharmaceutical preparation) and a solution containing 25 mg dichloromethotrexate in 3 mL DMSO. The method affords better than 99.5% destruction for the samples tested.

The residues produced by this method were tested for mutagenicity using *Salmonella typhimurium* strains TA1530, TA1535 and TA100 with and without metabolic activation. Mutagenic activity was detected only in the destruction products of pharmaceutical preparations of dichloromethotrexate, in which two to three times the background level of spontaneous revertants was observed when the maximal concentration that can be destroyed was tested in TA1530 strain.

For recommended applications of this method, see Methods Index, page 21.

2. PRINCIPLE

Destruction is effected by oxidation with potassium permanganate/sulfuric acid solution.

3. HAZARDS

3.1 *From methotrexate and dichloromethotrexate*

Although there is no unequivocal evidence of the carcinogenicity of methotrexate, this compound is teratogenic. No data concerning the carcinogenicity or teratogenicity of dichloromethotrexate were found in the literature. It is good laboratory practice to wear gloves even when handling compounds for which data on toxicity and carcinogenicity are incomplete.

A number of guidelines for the safe handling of antineoplastic agents have been published (Knowles & Virden, 1980; Davis, 1981; Harrison, 1981; Zimmerman *et al.*,

1981; Anderson *et al.*, 1982; National Institutes of Health 1982; Jones *et al.*, 1983; Solimando, 1983; Stolar *et al.*, 1983; National Study Commission on Cytotoxic Exposure, 1984; American Society of Hospital Pharmacists, 1985).

3.2 *Other hazards*

Concentrated sulfuric acid and sodium hydroxide are corrosive and should be handled with care.

Care should be taken in the preparation of solutions of potassium permanganate in sulfuric acid; never add solid potassium permanganate to concentrated sulfuric acid.

The dilution of concentrated sulfuric acid with water is an extremely exothermic reaction; always add the acid to the water, never the reverse, and remove heat by cooling in a cold-water bath.

Potassium permanganate is a strong oxidizing agent; care must be taken not to mix it with concentrated reducing agents.

In case of skin contact with corrosive chemicals, wash the skin with flowing water for at least 15 min.

4.   REAGENTS

4.1 *For destruction*

Potassium permanganate	Technical grade
Sulfuric acid (concentrated)	Specific gravity, 1.84 (about 18 mol/L); technical grade
Sulfuric acid solution	3 mol/L, aqueous (see Hazards, 3.2)
Potassium permanganate/sulfuric acid solution	To 100 ml of a 3 mol/L sulfuric acid solution, add 4.7 g solid potassium permanganate.

NOTE: The reagent should always be freshly prepared on the day of use.

Ascorbic acid or sodium bisulfite	Technical grade
Ascorbic acid or sodium bisulfite solution	$\simeq 50$ g/L, aqueous
Sodium hydroxide	Technical grade

Sodium hydroxide solution	$\simeq 2$ mol/L, aqueous ($\simeq 8$ g/ 100 mL)
Sodium carbonate	Technical grade

4.2 *For analysis*

Ascorbic acid	Analytical grade
Methanol	HPLC grade
Acetonitrile	HPLC grade
Water	Redistilled from glass
Tetrabutylammonium phosphate	Analytical grade
Phosphoric acid	Analytical grade
Tetrabutylammonium phosphate (solution)	5 mmol/L, aqueous (1.7 g/l), adjusted to pH 3.5 with phosphoric acid

5.   APPARATUS

Usual laboratory equipment and the following items: liquid chromatograph equipped with a reverse-phase ODS column and a UV detection system capable of measurement at 254 nm.

6.   PROCEDURE

Fifty mg of methotrexate or 10 mg of dichloromethotrexate (solid compound) dissolved in 10 mL of 3 mol/L sulfuric acid are destroyed by 0.5 g potassium permanganate in 1 h.

> NOTE: In the case of pharmaceutical preparations of dichloromethotrexate, up to 50 mg can be dissolved in 10 ml of 3 mol/L sulfuric acid and can be satisfactorily destroyed with 0.5 g of potassium permanganate.

6.1 *Solid compounds*

6.1.1   For each 50 mg methotrexate or about 10 mg dichloromethotrexate add 10 mL of 3 mol/L sulfuric acid.

6.1.2   Place on a magnetic stirrer, and add 0.5 g potassium permanganate per each 10 mL solution.

6.1.3   Continue stirring for 1 h.

6.1.4   If desired, check for completeness of degradation using the procedure described in Section 7.

6.1.5   Neutralize with 8 g/100 mL sodium hydroxide solution and discard.

6.2 *Aqueous solutions*

6.2.1   Dilute with water to obtain a maximum concentration of 5 mg/mL methotrexate or 1 mg/mL dichloromethotrexate.

6.2.2   Add slowly, with stirring, enough concentrated sulfuric acid to obtain a 3 mol/L solution (see 3.2, Hazards).

6.2.3   Proceed as in 6.1.2 to 6.1.5.

6.3 *Injectable pharmaceutical preparations*

NOTE: Solutions containing 2–5% glucose and 0.45% saline have been considered.

6.3.1   Dilute with water to obtain a maximum concentration of 2.5 mg/mL of either compound.

6.3.2   Add slowly, with stirring, enough concentrated sulfuric acid to obtain a 3 mol/L solution (see 3.2, Hazards).

6.3.3   Add 1 g potassium permanganate per each 10 mL solution and continue stirring for 1 h.

NOTE: To avoid frothing, add potassium permanganate in small increments.

6.3.4   Proceed as in 6.1.4 and 6.1.5.

6.4 *Solutions in volatile organic solvents*

6.4.1   Remove the solvent by evaporation, using a rotary evaporator, under reduced pressure.

6.4.2   Proceed as in 6.1.

6.5 *Solutions in DMSO or DMF*

6.5.1   Dilute with water to not more than 20% DMSO or DMF and to not more than 2.5 mg/mL of drug.

6.5.2   Proceed as in 6.3.2 to 6.3.4.

6.6 *Glassware*

6.6.1   Immerse in a freshly prepared solution of potassium permanganate/ sulfuric acid. Allow to react 1 h or more.

6.6.2   Clean the glass by immersion in a solution of ascorbic acid or sodium bisulfite.

6.7 *Spills of solid compounds*

6.7.1   Isolate the area, and put on suitable protective clothing.

6.7.2   Collect the solid, place it in a beaker and treat as in 6.1.

6.7.3   Rinse the area with an excess of 3 mol/L sulfuric acid solution. Take up the rinse with absorbent material.

6.7.4   Place the absorbent material in a beaker for inactivation (see 6.7.6).

6.7.5   If desired, check the surface for completeness of removal by wiping it with 0.1 mol/L sulfuric acid and analysing the wipe (see Section 7).

6.7.6   Cover the waste in the beaker with potassium permanganate/sulfuric acid solution. Allow to react for 1 h or more. If the purple colour fades, add more potassium permanganate.

6.7.7   Neutralize by addition of solid sodium carbonate. Discard.

6.8 *Spills of aqueous solutions or of injectable pharmaceutical preparations*

6.8.1   Isolate the area, and put on suitable protective clothing.

6.8.2   Take up the spill with absorbent material. Place the material in a beaker for inactivation.

6.8.3   Rinse the area with a 3 mol/L sulfuric acid solution and take up the rinse with an absorbent material. Place the absorbent material into the same beaker with the other waste.

6.8.4   Proceed as in 6.7.5 to 6.7.7.

6.9 *Spills of solutions in volatile organic solvents*

6.9.1   Isolate the area, and put on suitable protective clothing.

6.9.2   Allow the solvent to evaporate.

6.9.3   Proceed as in 6.7.3 to 6.7.7.

7.   ANALYSIS FOR COMPLETENESS OF DEGRADATION

7.1 Add ascorbic acid until the solution becomes colourless.

7.2 Analyse by HPLC, using the following conditions, or any other suitable HPLC reverse-phase chromatography system:

Column: 25 cm × 3.6 mm i.d., Partisil ODS-2 10 μm

Precolumn: 6.5 cm × 3.6 mm i.d., filled with CO:Pell ODS 30–38 μm

Eluant: For methotrexate, tetrabutylammonium phosphate solution:methanol (55:45)
For dichloromethotrexate, methanol:acetonitrile:tetrabutylammonium phosphate solution (11:22:66)

Flow rate: 1.5 mL/min

Injection volume: 50 μL

Detector: UV, 254 nm

8. SCHEMATIC REPRESENTATION OF PROCEDURE

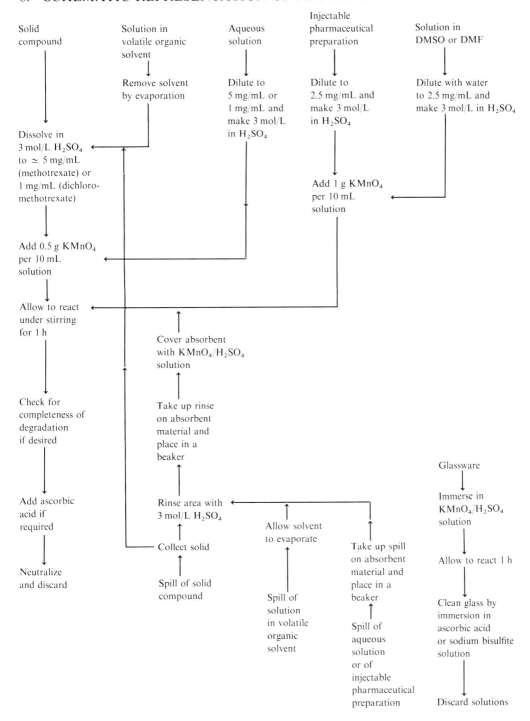

9. ORIGIN OF METHOD

Castegnaro, M., Michelon, J. & Brouet, I.
International Agency for Research on Cancer
150 Cours Albert Thomas
69372 Lyon Cedex 08, France

Contact point: M. CASTEGNARO

METHOD 3: DESTRUCTION OF METHOTREXATE USING AQUEOUS ALKALINE POTASSIUM PERMANGANATE

1. SCOPE AND FIELD OF APPLICATION

This method specifies the procedure for destruction of methotrexate in the following wastes: solid compound (6.1), aqueous solutions, including injectable pharmaceutical preparations (6.2), solutions in volatile organic solvents (6.3), glassware (6.4), spills of solid compound (6.5), spills of aqueous solutions (6.6) and spills of solutions in volatile organic solvents (6.7).

The method has been tested collaboratively using 50 mg of solid methotrexate and affords better than 99.5% degradation.

The residues produced by this method were tested for mutagenicity using *Salmonella typhimurium* strains TA1535, TA100 and UTH8414 with and without metabolic activation. No mutagenic activity was detected.

For recommended applications of this method, see Methods Index, page 21.

2. PRINCIPLE

Destruction of methotrexate is effected by oxidation with aqueous alkaline potassium permanganate.

3. HAZARDS

3.1 *From methotrexate*

Although there is no unequivocal evidence of the carcinogenicity of methotrexate, this compound is teratogenic. It is good laboratory practice to wear gloves when handling potentially hazardous compounds.

A number of guidelines for the safe handling of antineoplastic agents have been published (Knowles & Virden, 1980; Davis, 1981; Harrison, 1981; Zimmerman *et al.*, 1981; Anderson *et al.*, 1982; National Institutes of Health, 1982; Jones *et al.*, 1983; Solimando, 1983; Stolar *et al.*, 1983; National Study Commission on Cytotoxic Exposure, 1984; American Society of Hospital Pharmacists, 1985).

3.2 *Other hazards*

Sodium hydroxide and its solutions are corrosive and should be handled with care.

Potassium permanganate is a strong oxidizing agent; care must be taken not to mix it with concentrated reducing agents.

In case of skin contact with corrosive chemicals, wash the skin under flowing water for at least 15 min.

4. REAGENTS

4.1 *For destruction*

Potassium permanganate	Technical grade
Sodium hydroxide	Technical grade
Sodium bisulfite	Technical grade
Potassium permanganate solution	0.06 mol/L, aqueous (1 g/100 mL)
Sodium bisulfite solution	0.1 mol/L, aqueous (1 g/100 mL)
Sodium hydroxide solutions	1 mol/L, aqueous (4 g/100 mL) 2 mol/L, aqueous (8 g/100 mL)
Sodium hydroxide/potassium permanganate solution	1 g/100 mL potassium permanganate in 4 g/100 mL sodium hydroxide

4.2 *For analysis*

Methanol	Distilled in glass
Ammonium formate	Analytical grade
Water	Deionized, distilled
Formic acid	Analytical grade
Hydrochloric acid (concentrated)	Specific gravity, 1.19; 12 mol/L; analytical grade
Hydrochloric acid solution	$\simeq 1$ mol/L, aqueous
Sodium hydroxide	Analytical grade
Sodium hydroxide solution	0.1 mol/L, aqueous ($\simeq 0.4$ g/100 mL)

5. APPARATUS

Usual laboratory equipment and the following items: liquid chromatograph equipped with a reverse-phase ODS column and a UV detection system capable of measurement at 254 nm.

6. PROCEDURE

Fifty mg of methotrexate dissolved in 50 mL of 4 g/100 mL sodium hydroxide solution are destroyed by 5.5 mL of 1 g/100 mL potassium permanganate solution in 30 min.

6.1 *Solid compound*

6.1.1   Dissolve in 4 g/100 mL sodium hydroxide solution to obtain a concentration of not more than 1 mg/mL.

6.1.2   Add potassium permanganate solution until the purple colour persists for 30 min.

6.1.3   Add sodium bisulfite solution to the reaction mixture until the purple colour disappears.

6.1.4   If desired, check for degree of degradation using the procedure described in Section 7.

6.1.5   Discard.

6.2 *Aqueous solutions, including injectable pharmaceutical preparations*

6.2.1   Add an equal volume of 8 g/100 mL sodium hydroxide solution.

6.2.2   Proceed as in 6.1.2 to 6.1.5.

6.3 *Solutions in volatile organic solvents*

6.3.1   Estimate the amount of methotrexate to be degraded.

6.3.2   Remove the solvent by evaporation, using a rotary evaporator, under reduced pressure.

6.3.3   Proceed as in 6.1.

6.4 *Glassware*

6.4.1   Immerse in potassium permanganate/sodium hydroxide solution. Allow to react 30 min.

6.4.2   Clean the glass by immersion in sodium bisulfite solution.

6.5 *Spills of solid compound*

6.5.1   Isolate the area, and put on suitable protective clothing.

6.5.2   Collect the solid, place it in a beaker.

6.5.3   Rinse the area with 4 g/100 mL sodium hydroxide solution.

6.5.4   Take up the rinse with absorbent material; place material in same beaker as solid.

6.5.5   If desired, check the surface for completeness of removal by wiping it with absorbent material moistened with 0.1 mol/L sodium hydroxide solution and analysing the wipe (see Section 7).

6.5.6   Cover the waste in the beaker with potassium permanganate/sodium hydroxide solution and allow to react 30 min.

6.5.7   Discard.

6.6 *Spills of aqueous solutions*

6.6.1   Isolate the area, and put on suitable protective clothing.

6.6.2   Take up the spill with absorbent material. Place the material in a beaker and cover with alkaline potassium permanganate solution.

6.6.3   Proceed as in 6.5.3 to 6.5.7.

6.7 *Spills of solutions in volatile organic solvents*

6.7.1   Isolate the area, and put on suitable protective clothing.

6.7.2   Allow the solvent to evaporate.

6.7.3   Proceed as in 6.5.3 to 6.5.7.

7.   ANALYSIS FOR COMPLETENESS OF DEGRADATION

7.1 To an aliquot of solution to be analysed, add sodium bisulfite solution until colourless, then neutralize with 1 mol/L hydrochloric acid solution.

7.2 Analyse by HPLC, using the following conditions, or any other suitable HPLC chromatography system:

Column: Reverse-phase ODS, 25 cm $\times$ 3.9 mm i.d.

Eluant: 5 mmol/L ammonium formate, adjusted to pH 3.5 with formic acid: methanol (60:40)

Flow rate: 1 mL/min

Injection volume: 10 μl

Detector: UV, 254 nm

8.   SCHEMATIC REPRESENTATION OF PROCEDURE

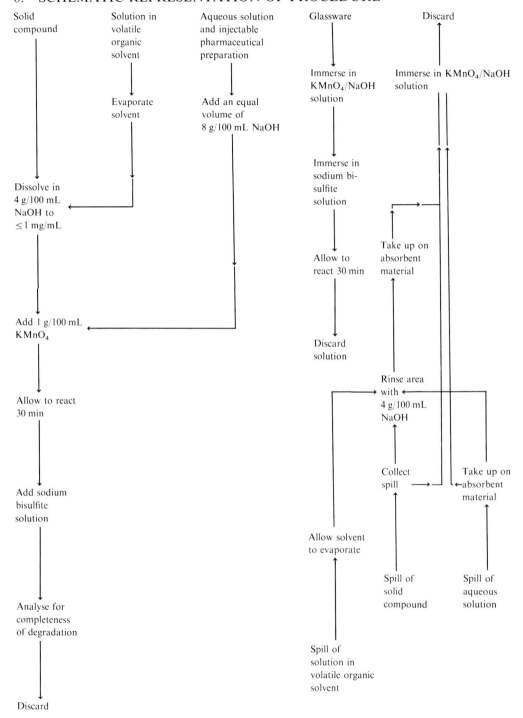

9. ORIGIN OF METHOD
   University of Texas System Cancer Center
   M.D. Anderson Hospital and Tumor Institute
   Departments of Pharmacy and Chemotherapy Research
   6723 Bertner Avenue
   Houston, Texas 77030, USA

   Contact point: J.A. BENVENUTO

METHOD 4: DESTRUCTION OF METHOTREXATE USING AQUEOUS SODIUM HYPOCHLORITE

1. SCOPE AND FIELD OF APPLICATION

This method specifies a procedure for the destruction of methotrexate in the following wastes: solid compound (6.1), aqueous solutions, including injectable pharmaceutical preparations (6.2), solutions in volatile organic solvents (6.3), glassware (6.4), spills of solid compound (6.5), spills of aqueous solutions and injectable pharmaceutical preparations (6.6) and spills of solutions in volatile organic solvents (6.7).

The method has been tested collaboratively using 50 mg of solid methotrexate and affords better than 99.5% degradation.

The residues produced by this method were tested for mutagenicity using *Salmonella typhymurium* strains TA1535, TA100 and UTH8414 with and without microsomal activation. No mutagenic activity was detected.

For recommended applications of this method, see Methods Index, page 21.

2. PRINCIPLE

Destruction of methotrexate is effected by oxidation with sodium hypochlorite.

3. HAZARDS

3.1 *From methotrexate*

Although there is no unequivocal evidence of the carcinogenicity of methotrexate, this compound is teratogenic. It is good laboratory practice to wear gloves when handling potentially hazardous compounds.

A number of guidelines for the safe handling of antineoplastic agents have been published (Knowles & Virden, 1980; Davis, 1981; Harrison, 1981; Zimmerman *et al.*,1981; Anderson *et al.*, 1982; National Institutes of Health, 1982; Jones *et al.*, 1983; Solimando, 1983; Stolar *et al.*, 1983; National Study Commission on Cytotoxic Exposure, 1984; American Society of Hospital Pharmacists, 1985).

3.2 *Other hazards*

Sodium hydroxide and its solutions are corrosive and should be handled with care.

Sodium hypochlorite is a strong oxidizing agent; care must be taken not to mix it with concentrated reducing agents.

In case of skin contact with corrosive chemicals, wash the skin under flowing water for at least 15 min.

4. REAGENTS

4.1 *For destruction*

Sodium hypochlorite solution	Commercial grade, 5% or 48°Cl
Sodium hydroxide	Technical grade
Sodium hydroxide solution	1 mol/L, aqueous (4 g/100 mL)

4.2 *For analysis*

Sodium bisulfite	Technical grade
Sodium bisulfite solution	0.1 mol/L, aqueous (1 g/100 mL)
Methanol	Distilled in glass
Ammonium formate	Analytical grade
Formic acid	Analytical grade
Water	Deionized, distilled
Hydrochloric acid (concentrated)	Specific gravity, 1.19; 12 mol/L, analytical grade
Hydrochloric acid solution	1 mol/L, aqueous

5. APPARATUS

Usual laboratory equipment and the following items: liquid chromatograph equipped with a reverse-phase ODS column and a UV detection system capable of measurement at 254 nm.

6. PROCEDURE

Fifty mg of methotrexate dissolved in 100 mL of 4 g/100 mL sodium hydroxide are destroyed by 4.6 mL of 5.25% sodium hypochlorite in 30 min.

NOTE 1: It must be remembered that solutions of sodium hypochlorite tend to deteriorate. It is therefore essential to check their active chlorine content. Note that the strength of sodium hypochlorite solutions may be given as weight/weight or weight/volume. This is an additional reason for estimating the concentration of available chlorine.

NOTE 2: Percent (%) available chlorine = mass of chlorine in grams liberated by acidifying 100 g of sodium hypochlorite solution. The available chlorine may also be expressed as °Cl, which corresponds to the volume of chlorine, in litres, liberated by one litre (liquid) or one kilogram (solid) of commercial bleach under treatment by hydrochloric acid, e.g., a 1 mol/L solution of hypochlorite corresponds to 22.4°Cl.

NOTE 3: The sodium hypochlorite solution used for this determination should contain not less than 25 g and not more than 30 g of active chlorine per litre. Assay: pipette 10.00 mL sodium hypochlorite solution into a 100-mL volumetric flask and fill to the mark with distilled water. Pipette 10 mL of the resulting solution into a conical flask containing 50 mL distilled water, 1 g potassium iodide and 12.5 mL acetic acid (2 mol/L). Rinse and titrate with 0.1 N sodium thiosulfate, using starch as indicator; 1 mL sodium thiosulfate (0.1 N) corresponds to 3.545 mg active chlorine.

6.1 *Solid compound*

6.1.1   Dissolve in 4 g/100 mL sodium hydroxide solution to obtain a concentration of not more than 50 mg/100 mL.

6.1.2   Estimate the amount of sodium hypochlorite solution required.

6.1.3   Add at least twice this estimated amount, i.e., $\simeq$ 10 mL sodium hypochlorite solution for each 50 mg methotrexate. Allow to react for 30 min.

6.1.4   If desired, check for completeness of degradation using the procedure described in Section 7.

6.1.5   Discard.

6.2 *Aqueous solutions, including injectable pharmaceutical preparations*

6.2.1   Estimate the amount of methotrexate to be degraded.

6.2.2   Proceed as in 6.1.2 to 6.1.5.

6.3 *Solutions in volatile organic solvents*

6.3.1   Estimate the amount of methotrexate to be degraded.

6.3.2   Remove the solvent by evaporation, using a rotary evaporator, under reduced pressure.

6.3.3   Proceed as in 6.1.

6.4 *Glassware*

Immerse in sodium hypochlorite solution. Allow to react 30 min. Discard.

6.5 *Spills of solid compound*

6.5.1   Isolate the area, and put on suitable protective clothing.

6.5.2   Collect the solid, place it in a beaker and treat as in 6.1.

6.5.3   Rinse the area with sodium hypochlorite solution and then with water.

6.5.4   Take up the rinse with absorbent material and discard.

6.5.5   If desired, check the surface for completeness of removal by wiping it with absorbent material moistened with 0.1 mol/L sodium hydroxide solution and analysing the wipe (see Section 7).

6.6 *Spills of aqueous solutions and injectable pharmaceutical preparations*

6.6.1   Isolate the area, and put on suitable protective clothing.

6.6.2   Take up on absorbent material. Place the material in a beaker.

6.6.3   Proceed as in 6.1.2 to 6.1.5.

6.7 *Spills of solutions in volatile organic solvents*

6.7.1   Isolate the area, and put on suitable protective clothing.

6.7.2   Allow the solvent to evaporate.

6.7.3   Proceed as in 6.5.3 to 6.5.5.

7.   ANALYSIS FOR COMPLETENESS OF DEGRADATION

7.1 To an aliquot of the solution to be analysed, add sodium bisulfite solution to reduce oxidant, then neutralize with 1 mol/L hydrochloric acid solution.

NOTE: Destruction of excess hypochlorite should always be performed in a fume cupboard, because chlorine is a by-product of the reaction.

7.2 Analyse by HPLC, using the following conditions, or any other suitable system:

Column: Reverse-phase ODS, 25 cm × 3.9 mm i.d.

Eluant: 5 mmol/L ammonium formate, pH 3.5 with formic acid:methanol (60:40)

Flow rate: 1 mL/min

Injection volume: 10 μL

Detector: UV, 254 nm

8.   SCHEMATIC REPRESENTATION OF PROCEDURE

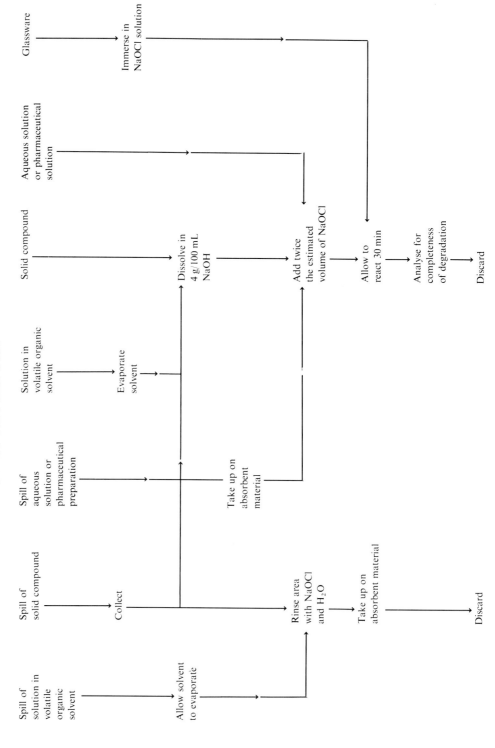

9. ORIGIN OF METHOD

    University of Texas System Cancer Center
    M.D. Anderson Hospital and Tumor Institute
    Departments of Pharmacy and Chemotherapy Research
    6723 Bertner Avenue
    Houston, Texas 77030, USA

    Contact point: J.A. BENVENUTO

METHOD 5: DESTRUCTION OF CYCLOPHOSPHAMIDE AND IFOSFAMIDE USING ALKALINE HYDROLYSIS IN THE PRESENCE OF DIMETHYLFORMAMIDE

1. SCOPE AND FIELD OF APPLICATION

This method specifies a procedure for the treatment of cyclophosphamide and ifosfamide in the following wastes: solid compounds (7.1), aqueous solutions and pharmaceutical solutions (7.2), solutions in dimethylformamide (DMF) (7.3), solutions in volatile organic solvents (7.4), solutions in dimethylsulfoxide (DMSO) (7.5), glassware (7.6), spills of solid compounds (7.7), spills of aqueous solutions or of solutions in DMF or DMSO (7.8) and spills of solutions in volatile organic solvents (7.9).

The method has been tested collaboratively using 100 mg solid ifosfamide and using a solution of 100 mg cyclophosphamide in 4 mL DMSO. The method affords better than 99% degradation for the samples tested.

The residues produced by this method were tested for mutagenicity using *Salmonella typhymurium* strains TA1530, TA1535 and TA100 with and without metabolic activation. No mutagenic activity was detected.

For recommended applications of this method, see Methods Index, page 21.

2. REFERENCES

Brooke, D., Scott, J.A. & Bequette, R.J. (1975) Effect of briefly heating cyclophosphamide solutions. *Am. J. Hosp. Pharm., 32,* 44–45

Friedman, O.M. (1967) Recent biologic and chemical studies of cyclophosphamide (NSC-26271). *Cancer Chemother. Rep., 51(6),* 327–333

3. PRINCIPLE

Destruction is effected by refluxing with a mixture of DMF and sodium hydroxide.

4. HAZARDS

4.1 *From cyclophosphamide or ifosfamide*

Cyclophosphamide is carcinogenic to humans, and ifosfamide has been shown to be carcinogenic to animals. Gloves must be worn for all operations involving the handling of these compounds or their solutions. Should gloves come into contact with solutions of these compounds, they should be changed as quickly as possible to reduce the risk of contact with the skin. The gloves should be discarded after use.

A number of guidelines for the safe handling of antineoplastic agents have been published (Knowles & Virden, 1980; Davis, 1981; Harrison, 1981; Zimmerman *et al.*, 1981; Anderson *et al.*, 1982; National Institutes of Health, 1982; Jones *et al.*, 1983, Solimando, 1983; Stolar *et al.*, 1983; National Study Commission on Cytotoxic Exposure, 1984; American Society of Hospital Pharmacists, 1985).

4.2 *Other hazards*

Hydrochloric acid and sodium hydroxide and their solutions are corrosive and should be handled with care.

DMF is an irritant, and skin contact should be avoided.

5. REAGENTS

5.1 *For destruction*

Sodium hydroxide	Technical grade
Sodium hydroxide solution	$\simeq 10$ mol/L, aqueous (40 g/100 mL) $\simeq 3$ mol/L, aqueous (12 g/100 mL)
DMF	Analytical grade
DMSO	Analytical grade
DMF: sodium hydroxide solution	Freshly prepared solution containing 2 volumes DMF and 1 volume of 12 g/100 mL sodium hydroxide

5.2 *For analysis*

Potassium dihydrogenphosphate (KH_2PO_4)	Analytical grade
Acetonitrile	HPLC grade
Water	Redistilled from glass
Hydrochloric acid	Specific gravity, 1.19; $\simeq 12$ mol/L, technical grade

Hydrochloric acid solution $\simeq$ 5 mol/L, aqueous

Phosphoric acid   Analytical grade

6. APPARATUS

Usual laboratory equipment and the following items: HPLC equipped with a reverse-phase ODS column and a UV detection system capable of measurement at 210 nm.

7. PROCEDURE

Ten mL of 12 g/100 mL sodium hydroxide are sufficient to destroy 100 mg cyclophosphamide or ifosfamide in 20 mL DMF when refluxed for 4 h.

7.1 *Solid compounds*

   7.1.1   For each 100 mg of sample, add 30 mL DMF/sodium hydroxide solution.

   7.1.2   Reflux for 4 h.

   7.1.3   If desired, check for completeness of degradation, using the procedure described in Section 8.

   7.1.4   Dilute with water and discard.

7.2 *Aqueous solutions and pharmaceutical solutions*

   7.2.1   Dilute with 40 g/100 mL sodium hydroxide solution to obtain a maximum content of 10 g/L cyclophosphamide and/or ifosfamide and a minimum concentration of 12 g/100 mL sodium hydroxide.

   7.2.2   Add 2 mL DMF for each mL of solution from 7.2.1.

   7.2.3   Proceed as in 7.1.2 to 7.1.4.

7.3 *Solutions in DMF*

   7.3.1   Estimate the amount of cyclophosphamide and/or ifosfamide to be degraded, and dilute, if necessary, with DMF to obtain not more than 5 g/L of drug.

   7.3.2   For each 2 mL of solution from 7.3.1, add 1 mL of 12 g/100 mL sodium hydroxide solution.

7.3.3   Proceed as in 7.1.2 to 7.1.4.

7.4 *Solutions in volatile organic solvents*

7.4.1   Estimate the amount of cyclophosphamide and/or ifosfamide to be degraded.

7.4.2   Remove the solvent by evaporation, using a rotary evaporator, under reduced pressure.

7.4.3   Proceed as in 7.1.

7.5 *Solutions in DMSO*

7.5.1   Estimate the amount of cyclophosphamide and/or ifosfamide to be destroyed and dilute, if necessary, with DMSO to obtain not more than 20 g/L of drug.

7.5.2   Add an equal volume of DMF and enough 12 g/100 mL sodium hydroxide solution to obtain a minimum concentration of 4 g/100 mL sodium hydroxide and a maximum concentration of not more than 5 g/L cyclophosphamide and/or ifosfamide.

7.5.3   Proceed as in 7.1.2 to 7.1.4.

7.6 *Glassware*

7.6.1   Rinse with two successive portions of 12 g/100 mL sodium hydroxide, then two successive portions of water (enough to wet all the glass). Drain completely between each rinse.

7.6.2   Treat rinses as in 7.2.

7.7 *Spills of solid compounds*

7.7.1   Isolate the area, and put on suitable protective clothing.

7.7.2   Collect the solid, place it in a beaker and treat as in 7.1.

7.7.3   Rinse the area with an excess of a solution of 12 g/100 mL sodium hydroxide.

7.7.4   Take up the rinse on absorbent material, and immerse the material in a freshly prepared DMF/sodium hydroxide solution.

7.7.5   Repeat steps 7.7.3 and 7.7.4.

7.7.6   If desired, check the surface for completeness of removal by wiping with absorbent material moistened with methanol and analysing the wipe (see Section 8).

7.7.7   Proceed as in 7.1.2 to 7.1.4.

7.8   *Spills of aqueous solutions or of solutions in DMF or DMSO*

7.8.1   Isolate the area, and put on suitable protective clothing.

7.8.2   Take up on absorbent material, and immerse the material in a freshly prepared DMF/sodium hydroxide solution.

7.8.3   Proceed as in 7.7.3 to 7.7.8.

7.9   *Spills of solutions in volatile organic solvents*

7.9.1   Isolate the area, and put on suitable protective clothing.

7.9.2   Allow the solvent to evaporate.

7.9.3   Proceed as in 7.7.3 to 7.7.8.

8.   ANALYSIS FOR COMPLETENESS OF DEGRADATION

8.1   Bring the pH of an aliquot of the sample to be analysed to 5–7 using 5 mol/L hydrochloric acid.

8.2   Analyse by HPLC, using the following conditions, or any other suitable HPLC reverse-phase chromatography system:

Column: 25 cm × 3.6 mm i.d., Partisil ODS-2 10 μm

Precolumn: 6.5 cm × 3.6 mm i.d., filled with CO:Pell ODS 30–38 μm

Solvent: Buffer 0.02 mol/L KH_2PO_4 adjusted to pH 4.5 with H_3PO_4:acetonitrile (65:35). Isocratic system

Flow rate: 1.5 mL/min

Injection volume: 50 μL

Detector: UV, 210 nm

9.   SCHEMATIC REPRESENTATION OF PROCEDURE

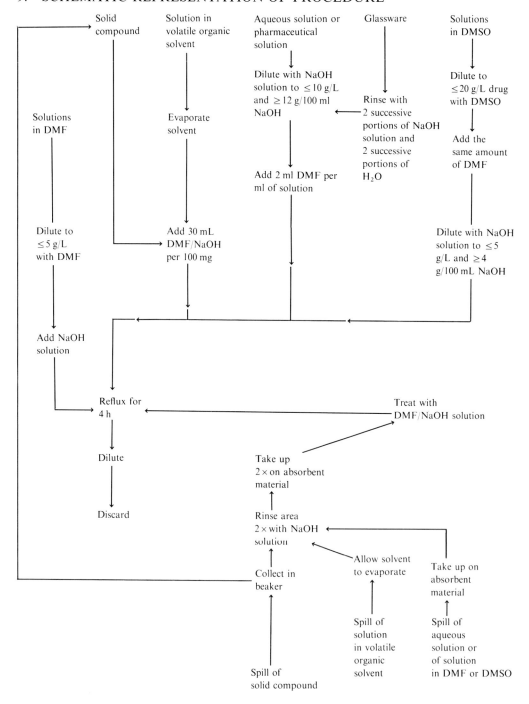

10. ORIGIN OF METHOD

Castegnaro, M., Michelon, J. & Brouet, I.
International Agency for Research on Cancer
150 Cours Albert Thomas
69372 Lyon Cedex 08, France

Contact point: M. CASTEGNARO

METHOD 6: DESTRUCTION OF CYCLOPHOSPHAMIDE USING ACID HYDROLYSIS FOLLOWED BY ADDITION OF SODIUM THIOSULFATE AND ALKALINE HYDROLYSIS

1. SCOPE AND FIELD OF APPLICATION

This method specifies a procedure for the destruction of cyclophosphamide in the following laboratory wastes: solid compound (6.1), aqueous solutions and injectable pharmaceutical preparations (6.2), solutions in dimethylformamide (DMF) and dimethylsulfoxide (DMSO) (6.3), solutions in volatile organic solvents (6.4), glassware (6.5), spills of solid compound (6.6), spills of aqueous solutions or of solutions in DMF or DMSO (6.7) and spills of solutions in volatile organic solvents (6.8).

The method has been tested collaboratively using 100 mg solid cyclophosphamide. The method affords better than 99% degradation for the samples tested.

The residues produced by this method were tested for mutagenicity using *Salmonella typhimurium* strains TA1530, TA1535 and TA100 with and without metabolic activation. No mutagenic activity was detected.

> NOTE: The method was also tested for the destruction of ifosfamide. Although chemical degradation was achieved, the residues possessed high mutagenic activity in each of the three strains tested. This method should therefore not be used to degrade ifosfamide.

For recommended applications of this method, see Methods Index, page 21.

2. PRINCIPLE

Destruction is effected by refluxing with hydrochloric acid and trapping the degradation products with sodium thiosulfate under alkaline conditions.

3. HAZARDS

3.1 *From cyclophosphamide*

Cyclophosphamide is carcinogenic to humans. Gloves must be worn for all operations involving the handling of this compound or its solutions. Should gloves come into contact with a solution of this compound, they should be changed as quickly as possible to reduce the risk of contact with the skin. The gloves should be discarded after use.

A number of guidelines for the safe handling of antineoplastic agents have been published (Knowles & Virden, 1980; Davis, 1981; Harrison, 1981; Zimmerman *et al.*,

1981; Anderson *et al.*,1982; National Institutes of Health, 1982; Jones *et al.*, 1983; Solimando, 1983; Stolar *et al.*, 1983; National Study Commission on Cytotoxic Exposure, 1984; American Society of Hospital Pharmacists, 1985).

3.2 *Other hazards*

Hydrochloric acid and sodium hydroxide and their solutions are corrosive and should be handled with care. All reactions must be carried out under a well-ventilated fume hood.

4. REAGENTS

4.1 *For destruction*

Sodium hydroxide	Technical grade
Sodium hydroxide solution	5 mol/L, aqueous (20 g/100 mL)
Sodium thiosulfate	Technical grade
Hydrochloric acid (concentrated)	Specific gravity, 1.19; $\simeq$ 12 mol/L; technical grade
Hydrochloric acid solution	1 and 2 mol/L, aqueous
pH paper	

4.2 *For analysis*

Potassium dihydrogenphosphate (KH_2PO_4)	Analytical grade
Acetonitrile	HPLC grade
Water	Redistilled from glass
Hydrochloric acid (concentrated)	Specific gravity, 1.19; 12 mol/L, analytical grade
Phosphoric acid	Analytical grade

5. APPARATUS

Usual laboratory equipment and the following items: HPLC equipped with a reverse-phase ODS column and a UV detection system capable of measurement at 210 nm.

6. PROCEDURE

A sample of 250 mg cyclophosphamide dissolved in 10 mL of 1 mol/L hydro-chloric acid solution is completely hydrolysed when refluxed for 1 h. After addition of 1.5 g sodium thiosulfate to the neutralized reaction mixture, the medium is made strongly alkaline with 20 g/100 mL sodium hydroxide solution and the reaction allowed to proceed for 1 h.

6.1 *Solid compound*

6.1.1   For each 250 mg of sample, add 10 mL of 1 mol/L hydrochloric acid solution.

6.1.2   Reflux for 1 h. Allow to cool to room temperature.

6.1.3   Add 20 g/100 mL sodium hydroxide solution until a pH of about 6 is obtained. Allow to cool to room temperature.

6.1.4   Add 1.5 g sodium thiosulfate for each 250 mg cyclophosphamide and make strongly alkaline with 20 g/100 mL sodium hydroxide solution.

6.1.5   Allow to react for 1 h.

6.1.6   If desired, check for completeness of degradation, using the procedure described in Section 7.

6.1.7   Dilute with water and discard.

6.2 *Aqueous solutions and injectable pharmaceutical preparations*

6.2.1   Dilute if necessary to obtain a maximum cyclophosphamide content of 25 g/L and add concentrated hydrochloric acid to obtain a 1 mol/L hydrochloric acid solution.

6.2.2   Proceed as in 6.1.2 to 6.1.7.

6.3 *Solutions in DMF or DMSO*

6.3.1   Dilute with water, if necessary, to obtain a maximum content of cyclophosphamide of 50 g/L. Add an equal volume of 2 mol/L hydrochloric acid solution.

6.3.2   Proceed as in 6.1.2 to 6.1.7.

6.4 *Solutions in volatile organic solvents*

6.4.1   Estimate the amount of cyclophosphamide to be degraded.

6.4.2   Remove the solvent by evaporation, using a rotary evaporator, under reduced pressure.

6.4.3   Proceed as in 6.1.

6.5 *Glassware*

6.5.1   Rinse with four successive portions of 1 mol/L hydrochloric acid solution (enough to wet all the glass). Drain completely between each rinse.

6.5.2   Treat rinses as in 6.1.2 to 6.1.7.

6.6 *Spills of solid compound*

6.6.1   Isolate the area, and put on suitable protective clothing.

6.6.2   Collect the solid and place in a beaker.

6.6.3   Rinse the area with four successive portions of enough 1 mol/L hydrochloric acid solution to wet it. Take up each rinse on absorbent material. Place material in the beaker containing the solid from 6.6.2.

6.6.4   If desired, check the surface for completeness of removal by wiping with absorbent material moistened with methanol and analysing the wipe (see Section 7).

6.6.5   Cover the contents of the beaker from 6.6.2 and 6.6.3 with 1 mol/L hydrochloric acid solution.

6.6.6   Proceed as in 6.1.2 to 6.1.5.

6.6.7   Discard.

6.7 *Spills of aqueous solutions or of solutions in DMF or DMSO*

6.7.1   Isolate the area, and put on suitable protective clothing.

6.7.2   Take up on absorbent material; transfer the material to a beaker and cover it with 1 mol/L hydrochloric acid solution.

6.7.3   Rinse the area with four successive portions of enough 1 mol/L hydrochloric acid solution to wet it.

6.7.4   If desired, check the surface for completeness of removal by wiping with an absorbent material moistened with methanol and analysing the wipe (see Section 7).

6.7.5   Take up each rinse on absorbent material, and immediately immerse the material in the beaker containing the residues from 6.7.2.

6.7.6   Proceed as in 6.1.2 to 6.1.5.

6.8 *Spills of solutions in volatile organic solvents*

6.8.1   Isolate the area, and put on suitable protective clothing.

6.8.2   Allow the solvent to evaporate.

6.8.3   Proceed as in 6.6.3 to 6.6.7.

7. ANALYSIS FOR COMPLETENESS OF DEGRADATION

7.1 Bring the pH of an aliquot of the sample to be analysed to pH 5–7 using concentrated hydrochloric acid.

7.2 Analyse by HPLC, using the following conditions, or any other suitable HPLC reverse-phase chromatography system:

Column: 25 cm × 3.6 mm i.d., Partisil ODS-2 10 μm

Precolumn: 6.5 cm × 3.6 mm i.d., filled with CO:Pell ODS 30–38 μm

Solvent: Buffer 0.02 mol/L KH_2PO_4 adjusted to pH 4.5 with H_3PO_4:acetonitrile (65:35). Isocratic system. $R_T \simeq 8$ min

Flow rate: 1.5 mL/min

Injection volume: 50 μL

Detector: UV, 210 nm

8.   SCHEMATIC REPRESENTATION OF PROCEDURE

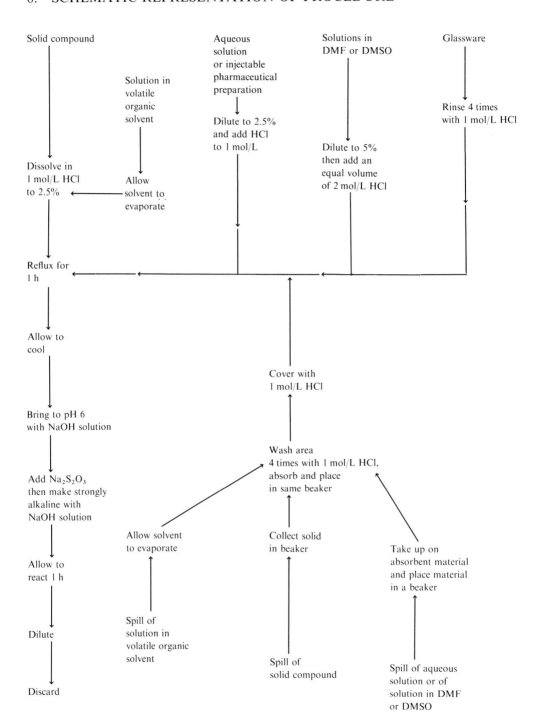

9.   ORIGIN OF METHOD

Ludeman, S. & Zon, G.
The Catholic University of America
Department of Chemistry
Washington DC 20064, USA

Brouet, I. & Michelon, J. (for testing of residues)
International Agency for Research on Cancer
150 Cours Albert Thomas
69372 Lyon Cedex 08, France

Contact point: S. LUDEMAN and G. ZON

METHOD 7: DESTRUCTION OF VINCRISTINE SULFATE AND VINBLASTINE SULFATE USING POTASSIUM PERMANGANATE/SULFURIC ACID

1. SCOPE AND FIELD OF APPLICATION

This method specifies a procedure for the destruction of vincristine sulfate and vinblastine sulfate in the following wastes: solid compounds (6.1), aqueous solutions (6.2), solutions in volatile organic solvents (6.3), solutions in dimethylformamide (DMF) or dimethylsulfoxide (DMSO) (6.4), pharmaceutical preparations (6.5), glassware (6.6), spills of solid compounds (6.7), spills of aqueous solutions or of solutions of pharmaceutical preparations (6.8) and spills of solutions in volatile organic solvents (6.9).

The method has been tested collaboratively with 1 mg vincristine sulfate (pharmaceutical preparation) and with a solution of 10 mg vinblastine sulfate in 2 ml DMSO. The method affords better than 99% degradation for the samples tested.

The residues of destruction of pharmaceutical preparations dissolved in water, DMF or DMSO were tested for mutagenicity using *Salmonella typhimurium* strains TA1535, TA98 and TA100 with and without metabolic activation. No mutagenic activity was detected.

2. PRINCIPLE

Destruction is effected by oxidation with a solution of potassium permanganate in sulfuric acid.

3. HAZARDS

3.1 *From vincristine sulfate and vinblastine sulfate*

Vincristine sulfate and vinblastine sulfate can induce teratogenic effects and embryolethality in several animal species. Appropriate precautions, e.g., working with gloves, must be taken when handling these compounds or their solutions.

A number of guidelines for the safe handling of antineoplastic agents have been published (Knowles & Virden, 1980; Davis, 1981; Harrison, 1981; Zimmerman *et al.*, 1981; Anderson *et al.*, 1982; National Institutes of Health, 1982; Jones *et al.*, 1983; Solimando, 1983; Stolar *et al.*, 1983; National Study Commission on Cytotoxic Exposure, 1984; American Society of Hospital Pharmacists, 1985).

3.2 *Other hazards*

Concentrated sulfuric acid and sodium hydroxide are corrosive and should be handled with care.

Care should be taken in the preparation of solutions of potassium permanganate in sulfuric acid; never add solid potassium permanganate to concentrated sulfuric acid.

The dilution of concentrated sulfuric acid with water is an extremely exothermic reaction; always add the acid to the water, never the reverse, and remove heat by cooling in a cold-water bath.

Potassium permanganate is a strong oxidizing agent; care must be taken not to mix it with concentrated reducing agents.

In case of skin contact with corrosive chemicals, wash the skin with flowing water for at least 15 min.

4.   REAGENTS

4.1 *For destruction*

Potassium permanganate	Technical grade
Sulfuric acid (concentrated)	Specific gravity, 1.84 (about 18 mol/L); technical grade
Sulfuric acid solution	$\simeq$ 3 mol/L, aqueous (see Hazards, 3.2)
Potassium permanganate/sulfuric acid solution	To 100 mL of a 3 mol/L sulfuric acid solution, add 4.7 g solid potassium permanganate.

NOTE: The reagent should always be freshly prepared on the day of use.

Ascorbic acid or sodium bisulfite	Technical grade
Ascorbic acid or sodium bisulfite solution	50 g/L, aqueous
Sodium hydroxide	Technical grade
Sodium hydroxide solution	$\simeq$ 2 mol/L, aqueous ($\simeq$ 8 g/100 mL)
Sodium carbonate	Technical grade

4.2 *For analysis*

Ascorbic acid	Analytical grade

Tetrabutylammonium phosphate	Analytical grade
Tetrabutylammonium phosphate solution	5 mmol/L, aqueous (1.7 g/100 mL), adjusted to pH 3.5 with phosphoric acid
Phosphoric acid	Analytical grade
Acetonitrile	HPLC grade
Tetrahydrofuran	HPLC grade
Water	Redistilled from glass

5. APPARATUS

Usual laboratory equipment and the following items: liquid chromatograph equipped with a reverse phase ODS column, and a UV detection system capable of measurement at 254 nm.

6. PROCEDURE

Ten mg of vincristine sulfate or vinblastine sulfate in 10 mL of 3 mol/L sulfuric acid solution are completely destroyed by 0.5 g potassium permanganate in 2 h.

6.1 *Solid compounds*

6.1.1   Estimate the amount of drug to be destroyed, and dissolve in 3 mol/L sulfuric acid solution to obtain a maximum content of 1 mg/mL.

6.1.2   Place flask on a magnetic stirrer; add 0.5 g potassium permanganate per 10 mL of solution from 6.1.1.

6.1.3   Continue stirring for 2 h or more.

6.1.4   If desired, check for completeness of destruction using the method described in Section 7.

6.1.5   Neutralize with 8 g/100 mL sodium hydroxide solution, and discard.

6.2 *Aqueous solutions*

6.2.1   Estimate the amount of drug to be destroyed, and dilute, if necessary, to a maximum content of 1 mg/mL.

6.2.2   Add slowly, with stirring, enough concentrated sulfuric acid to obtain a 3 mol/L solution, and allow to cool to room temperature (see 3.2, Hazards).

6.2.3   Proceed as in 6.1.2 to 6.1.5.

6.3 *Solutions in volatile organic solvents (including methanol and ethanol)*

6.3.1   Estimate the amount of drug to be destroyed.

6.3.2   Remove solvent by evaporation, using a rotary evaporator under reduced pressure.

6.3.3   Proceed as in 6.1.2 to 6.1.5.

6.4 *Solutions in DMF or DMSO*

6.4.1   Dilute with water to obtain a maximum concentration of 20% solvent and not more than 1 mg/mL of drug.

6.4.2   Add slowly, with stirring, enough concentrated sulfuric acid to obtain a concentration of 3 mol/L and allow to cool to room temperature (see 3.2, Hazards).

6.4.3   Place flask on a magnetic stirrer; gradually add 1 g potassium permanganate per 10 mL of solution.

NOTE: To avoid frothing, add the potassium permanganate in small increments.

6.4.4   Proceed as in 6.1.3 to 6.1.5.

6.5 *Pharmaceutical preparations*

NOTE 1: The following preparation was investigated: 1 mg of compound + 1.275 mg methyl *para*-hydroxybenzoate + 1.225 propyl *para*-hydroxybenzoate + 100 mg mannitol.

6.5.1   Estimate the amount of drug to be destroyed, and dissolve in 3 mol/L sulfuric acid solution to obtain a maximum content of 0.1 mg/mL.

6.5.2   Place on a magnetic stirrer; gradually add 0.5 g potassium permanganate per 10 mL of solution.

NOTE 2: To avoid frothing, add the potassium permanganate in small increments.

6.5.3   Proceed as in 6.1.3 to 6.1.5.

6.6 *Glassware*

6.6.1   Immerse in a freshly prepared solution of potassium permanganate/
sulfuric acid. Allow to react 2 h or more.

6.6.2   Clean the glass by immersion in a solution of ascorbic acid or sodium
bisulfite.

6.7 *Spills of solid compounds*

6.7.1   Isolate the area, and put on suitable protective clothing.

6.7.2   Collect the solid compound; place it in beaker.

6.7.3   Rinse the area with water. Take up the rinse on absorbent material, and
place the material in the beaker from 6.7.2.

6.7.4   If desired, check the surface for completeness of removal by wiping it
with absorbent material moistened with water and analysing the wipe
(see Section 7).

6.7.5   Cover the contents of the beaker from 6.7.3 with potassium permanga-
nate/sulfuric acid solution. Allow to react for 2 h. If the purple colour
fades, add more potassium permanganate.

6.7.6   Discard

6.8 *Spills of aqueous solutions or of solutions of pharmaceutical preparations*

6.8.1   Isolate the area, and put on suitable protective clothing.

6.8.2   Take up with absorbent material; place material in a beaker. Rinse the
area with water. Take up rinse with absorbent material, and place
material in the same beaker.

6.8.3   Proceed as in 6.7.4 to 6.7.6.

6.9 *Spills of solutions in volatile organic solvents*

6.9.1   Isolate the area and put on suitable protective clothing.

6.9.2   Allow the solvent to evaporate.

6.9.3   Proceed as in 6.7.3 to 6.7.6.

7.   ANALYSIS FOR COMPLETENESS OF DEGRADATION

7.1 Add ascorbic acid until the solution becomes colourless.

7.2 Analyse by HPLC, using the following conditions, or any other suitable system:

Column: 25 cm × 3.6 mm i.d., Partisil ODS-2 10 μm

Precolumn: 65 mm × 3.6 mm i.d., filled with CO:Pell ODS 30–38 μm

Solvent: Isocratic system. Tetrabutylammonium phosphate solution:aceto-
nitrile:tetrahydrofuran (54:26:20)

Flow rate: 1.5 mL/min

Injection volume: 50 μL

Detector: UV, 254 nm

8. SCHEMATIC REPRESENTATION OF PROCEDURE

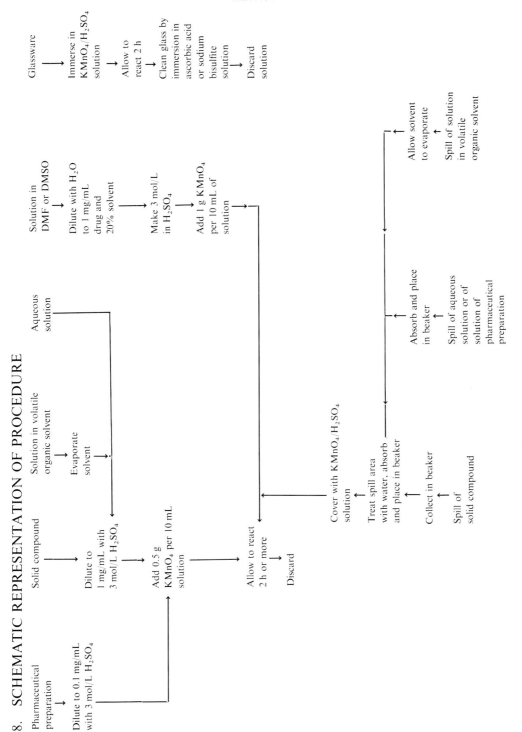

9. ORIGIN OF METHOD

Castegnaro, M., Michelon, J. & Brouet, I.
International Agency for Research on Cancer
150 Cours Albert Thomas
69372 Lyon Cedex 08, France

Contact point: M. CASTEGNARO

METHOD 8: DESTRUCTION OF 6-THIOGUANINE AND 6-MERCAPTOPURINE USING POTASSIUM PERMANGANATE/SULFURIC ACID

1. SCOPE AND FIELD OF APPLICATION

This method specifies a procedure for the destruction of 6-thioguanine and 6-mercaptopurine in the following wastes: solid compounds (6.1), aqueous solutions (6.2), solutions in volatile organic solvents (6.3), solutions in dimethylformamide (DMF) or dimethylsulfoxide (DMSO) (6.4), pharmaceutical preparations (6.5), glass-ware (6.6) and spills (6.7).

The method has been tested collaboratively with 20 mg solid 6-thioguanine and with a solution of 6-mercaptopurine (40 mg in 6 mL DMF). The method affords better than 99.5% destruction for the samples tested.

The residues produced by this method were tested for mutagenicity using *Salmonella typhimurium* strains TA1535, TA98 and TA100 with and without metabolic activation. No mutagenic activity was detected.

2. PRINCIPLE

Destruction is effected by oxidation with a solution of potassium permanganate in sulfuric acid.

3. HAZARDS

3.1 *From 6-mercaptopurine*

6-Mercaptopurine was shown to be mutagenic without metabolic activation in *Salmonella typhimurium* tester strains *his* G46 and TA1535 and must be handled with care. It is good laboratory practice to wear gloves when handling potentially hazard-ous compounds.

A number of guidelines for the safe handling of antineoplastic agents have been published (Knowles & Virden, 1980; Davis, 1981; Harrison, 1981; Zimmerman *et al.*, 1981; Anderson *et al.*, 1982; National Institutes of Health, 1982; Jones *et al.*, 1983; Solimando, 1983; Stolar *et al.*, 1983; National Study Commission on Cytotoxic Exposure, 1984; American Society of Hospital Pharmacists, 1985).

3.2 *Other hazards*

Concentrated sulfuric acid and potassium hydroxide are corrosive and should be handled with care.

Care should be taken in the preparation of solutions of potassium permanganate in sulfuric acid; never add solid potassium permanganate to concentrated sulfuric acid.

The dilution of concentrated sulfuric acid with water is an extremely exothermic reaction; always add the acid to the water, never the reverse, and remove heat by cooling in a cold water bath.

Potassium permanganate is a strong oxidizing agent; care must be taken not to mix it with concentrated reducing agents.

In case of skin contact with corrosive chemicals, wash the skin with flowing water for at least 15 min.

4. REAGENTS

4.1 *For destruction*

Potassium permanganate	Technical grade
Sulfuric acid (concentrated)	Specific gravity, 1.84 (about 18 mol/L); technical grade
Sulfuric acid solution	$\simeq$ 3 mol/L, aqueous (see 3.2, Hazards)
Potassium permanganate/sulfuric acid solution	To 100 mL of a 3 mol/L sulfuric acid solution, add 4.7 g solid potassium permanganate

NOTE: The reagent should always be freshly prepared on the day of use.

Ascorbic acid or sodium bisulfite	Technical grade
Ascorbic acid or sodium bisulfite solutions	$\simeq$ 50 g/L, aqueous
Sodium hydroxide	Technical grade
Sodium hydroxide solution	$\simeq$ 2 mol/L, aqueous ($\simeq$ 8 g/ 100 mL)
Sodium carbonate	Technical grade

4.2 *For analysis*

Ascorbic acid	Analytical grade

Potassium dihydrogenphosphate (KH$_2$PO$_4$)	Analytical grade
KH$_2$PO$_4$ solution	0.02 mol/L, aqueous
Water	Redistilled from glass
Acetonitrile	HPLC grade
Sodium hydroxide	Analytical grade
Sodium hydroxide solution	0.1 mol/L, aqueous (0.4 g/ 100 mL)

5. APPARATUS

Usual laboratory equipment and the following items: liquid chromatograph equipped with a reverse-phase ODS column and a UV spectrophotometer capable of measurement at 340 nm.

6. PROCEDURE

Eighteen mg of 6-thioguanine or 6-mercaptopurine dissolved in 20 mL of 3 mol/L sulfuric acid solution are destroyed by 0.13 g potassium permanganate in 10–12 h.

6.1 *Solid compounds*

6.1.1   Dissolve in 3 mol/L sulfuric acid to obtain a maximum concentration of 900 mg/L.

6.1.2   Place flask on a magnetic stirrer; add 0.5 g potassium permanganate per 80 mL of solution from 6.1.1.

6.1.3   Allow to react overnight.

6.1.4   If desired, check for completeness of destruction using the method described in Section 7.

6.1.5   Neutralize with 8 g/100 mL sodium hydroxide solution, and discard.

6.2 *Aqueous solutions*

6.2.1   If necessary, dilute with water to obtain a maximum concentration of 900 mg/L.

6.2.2   Add slowly, with stirring, enough concentrated sulfuric acid to obtain a 3 mol/L solution, and allow to cool to room temperature (see 3.2, Hazards).

6.2.3   Proceed as in 6.1.2 to 6.1.5.

6.3 *Solutions in volatile organic solvents*

6.3.1   Estimate the amount of compound to be destroyed.

6.3.2   Remove solvent by evaporation, using a rotary evaporator under reduced pressure.

6.3.3   Proceed as in 6.1.

6.4 *Solutions in DMF or DMSO*

6.4.1   Dilute with water to obtain a maximum concentration of 20% solvent and not more than 900 mg/L of drug.

6.4.2   Add slowly, with stirring, enough concentrated sulfuric acid to obtain a 3 mol/L solution, and allow to cool to room temperature (see 3.2, Hazards).

6.4.3   Place flask on a magnetic stirrer; gradually add 4 g potassium permanganate per 80 mL of solution.

NOTE: To avoid frothing, add the potassium permanganate in small increments.

6.4.4   Proceed as in 6.1.3 to 6.1.5.

6.5 *Pharmaceutical preparations*

6.5.1   Oral preparations

          6.5.1.1 Dissolve in 3 mol/L sulfuric acid.

          6.5.1.2 Proceed as in 6.4.3 – 6.4.4.

6.5.2   Parenteral solutions

          Two preparations were tested: 7.5 mg 6-thioguanine in 50 mL of 5% dextrose solution; and 10 mg 6-mercaptopurine in 10 mL of 5% dextrose solution: Proceed as in 6.4.2 to 6.4.4.

6.6 *Glassware*

6.6.1   Immerse in a freshly prepared solution of potassium permanganate/sulfuric acid. Allow to react 10–12 h.

6.6.2   Clean the glass by immersion in a solution of ascorbic acid or sodium bisulfite.

6.7 *Spills*

6.7.1   Isolate the area, and put on suitable protective clothing.

6.7.2   Collect the solid, or take up the liquid on absorbent material, and place the material in a beaker.

6.7.3   Rinse the area with 0.1 mol/L sulfuric acid. Take up the rinse with absorbent material, and place the material in the beaker from 6.7.2.

6.7.4   If desired, check the surface for completeness of removal by wiping it with absorbent material moistened with 0.1 mol/L sodium hydroxide solution and analysing the wipe (see Section 7).

6.7.5   Cover the contents of the beaker from 6.7.3 with 3 mol/L sulfuric acid and add, with stirring, an excess of potassium permanganate. Allow to react overnight.

NOTE: At the end of this period, some purple colour should remain; if not, add more potassium permanganate and continue to react.

6.7.6   Discard.

7. ANALYSIS FOR COMPLETENESS OF DEGRADATION

Several methods for the analysis of 6-thioguanine or 6-mercaptopurine are available in the literature. The following method may be used:

7.1 Add ascorbic acid until the solution becomes colourless.

7.2 Analyse by HPLC, using the following conditions:

Column: 25 cm × 3.6 mm i.d., Partisil ODS-2 10 µm

Precolumn: 6.5 cm × 3.6 mm i.d., filled with CO:Pell ODS 30–38 µm

Eluant: 0.02 mol/L KH_2PO_4:acetonitrile (98:2)

Flow rate: 1.5 mL/min

Injection volume: 50 µL

Detector: UV, 340 nm

8.   SCHEMATIC REPRESENTATION OF PROCEDURE

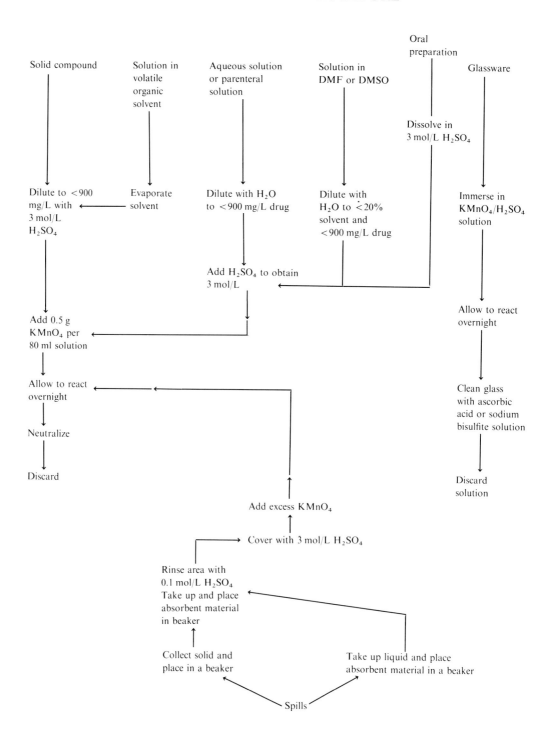

9. ORIGIN OF METHOD
    Dr J. Barek
    Department of Analytical Chemistry
    Charles University
    Albertov 2030
    12840 Prague 2, Czechoslovakia

    Castegnaro, M., Michelon, J. & Brouet, I.
    International Agency for Research on Cancer
    150 Cours Albert Thomas
    69372 Lyon Cedex 08, France

    Contact point: J. BAREK

METHOD 9: DESTRUCTION OF CISPLATIN BY REDUCTION WITH ZINC POWDER

1. SCOPE AND FIELD OF APPLICATION

This method specifies a procedure for the destruction of cisplatin in the following wastes: solid compound (6.1), aqueous solutions and injectable pharmaceutical preparations (6.2), solutions in water-miscible organic solvents (6.3) and glassware (6.4).

The method has been tested collaboratively using 30 mg cisplatin; it affords $\simeq 99\%$ destruction.

The residue produced by this method was tested for mutagenicity using *Salmonella typhimurium* strains TA98, TA100 and TA1535 with and without metabolic activation. No mutagenic activity was detected.

For recommended applications of this procedure, see Methods Index, page 22.

2. PRINCIPLE

Destruction is effected by reduction of cisplatin to elemental platinum with zinc powder under acidic conditions.

3. HAZARDS

3.1 *From cisplatin*

Cisplatin is probably carcinogenic to humans, and appropriate precautions, such as wearing gloves when handling the compound or its solutions, should be taken.

A number of guidelines for the safe handling of antineoplastic agents have been published (Knowles & Virden, 1980; Davis, 1981; Harrison, 1981; Zimmerman *et al.*, 1981; Anderson *et al.*, 1982; National Institutes of Health, 1982; Jones *et al.*, 1983; Solimando, 1983; Stolar *et al.*, 1983; National Study Commission on Cytotoxic Exposure, 1984; American Society of Hospital Pharmacists, 1985).

3.2 *Other hazards*

Concentrated sulfuric acid and sodium hydroxide are corrosive and should be handled with care.

The dilution of concentrated sulfuric acid with water is an extremely exothermic reaction; always add acid to the water, never the reverse, and remove heat by cooling in a cold-water bath.

In case of skin contact with corrosive chemicals, wash the skin with flowing water for at least 15 min.

4. REAGENTS

4.1 *For destruction*

Sulfuric acid (concentrated)	Specific gravity, 1.84 (about 18 mol/L); technical grade
Zinc powder	Technical grade
Sodium hydroxide	Technical grade
Sulfuric acid solution	$\simeq 2$ mol/L and $\simeq 4$ mol/L, aqueous (see Hazards, 3.2)
Sodium hydroxide solution	$\simeq 2$ mol/L, aqueous ($\simeq 8$ g/100 mL)

4.2 *For analysis*

Water	Redistilled from glass
Heptane	UV grade
Isopropanol	UV grade
Chloroform	Analytical grade
Chloroform	Water-saturated
Sodium nitrate	Analytical grade
Sodium nitrate solution	Saturated, aqueous
Sodium diethyldithiocarbamate	Analytical grade
Sodium hydroxide	Analytical grade
Sodium hydroxide solution	0.1 mol/L, aqueous (0.4 g/100 mL)
Sodium diethyldithiocarbamate solution	10% in 0.1 mol/L sodium hydroxide solution

5.   APPARATUS

Usual laboratory equipment and the following items:

Sintered glass funnel   Porosity 4 or similar

Atomic absorption spectrophotometer with platinum lamp

or

Liquid chromatograph equipped with a CN bonded phase column and a UV detection system capable of measurement at 254 nm.

6.   PROCEDURE

Thirty mg of cisplatin dissolved in 50 mL of 2 mol/L sulfuric acid solution are destroyed by 1.5 g zinc powder in 10–12 h.

6.1 *Solid compound*

6.1.1   Dissolve in 2 mol/L sulfuric acid solution to achieve a maximum concentration of 0.6 mg/mL.

6.1.2   Place flask on a magnetic stirrer; add 3 g zinc powder per 100 mL of solution from 6.1.1.

6.1.3   Stir overnight.

6.1.4   If desired, check for completeness of destruction using the method described in Section 7.

6.1.5   Neutralize with a 8 g/100 mL sodium hydroxide solution.

6.1.6   Discard.

6.2 *Aqueous solutions and injectable pharmaceutical preparations*

NOTE: Solutions in 5% dextrose or 0.9% saline were considered.

6.2.1   Dilute with water to obtain a maximum concentration of 0.6 mg/mL.

6.2.2   Add slowly, with stirring, enough concentrated sulfuric acid to obtain a 2 mol/L solution, and allow to cool to room temperature (see 3.2, Hazards).

6.2.3   Proceed as in 6.1.2 to 6.1.6.

6.3 *Solutions in water-miscible organic solvents*

    6.3.1   Add an equal volume of 4 mol/L sulfuric acid solution, or more if necessary, to achieve a maximum concentration of 0.6 mg/mL of drug.

    6.3.2   Proceed as in 6.1.2 to 6.1.6.

6.4 *Glassware*

    6.4.1   Rinse at least four times with enough water to completely wet the glass.

    6.4.2   Treat rinses as in 6.2.

7. ANALYSIS FOR COMPLETENESS OF DEGRADATION

7.1 By atomic absorption spectrophotometry

    7.1.1   Remove unreacted zinc powder by filtering through a sintered glass funnel; collect filtrate.

    7.1.2   To 2-mL fractions of filtrate, add 20, 40, 60, 80 or 100 μL of a 2 mol/L cisplatin solution.

    7.1.3   Determine platinum II, using the following conditions:
– acetylene-air flame
– band width, 0.5 nm
– wavelength, 260 nm
– Pt lamp

7.2 By HPLC

    7.2.1   Transfer a 9-mL aliquot of residual solution to a capped centrifuge tube. Add 1 mL sodium diethyldithiocarbamate solution and 1 mL sodium nitrate solution.

    7.2.2   Shake, and allow to react 1 h at room temperature.

    7.2.3   Add 1 mL of water-saturated chloroform to the tube from 7.2.1, and shake.

    7.2.4   Centrifuge for 5 min at 1200 $\times$ *g*; mix in a Vortex mixer, and centrifuge again for another 10 min.

    7.2.5   Discard aqueous layer and emulsion.

    7.2.6   Analyse, using the following conditions:

Column: 30 cm × 3.6 mm i.d., μ Bondapack CN

Eluant: Heptane:isopropanol (82:18)

Flow rate: 2 mL/min

Injection volume: 30 μL

Detector: UV, 254 nm

8. SCHEMATIC REPRESENTATION OF PROCEDURE

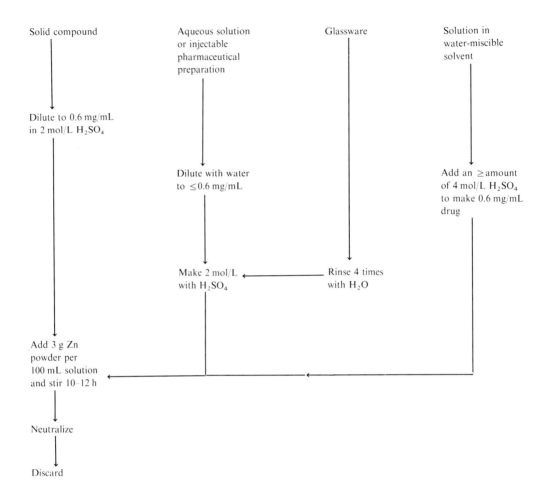

9.   ORIGIN OF METHOD

Dr J. Barek
Department of Analytical Chemistry
Charles University
Albertov 2030
12840 Prague 2, Czechoslovakia

Brouet, I. & Castegnaro, M. (for testing of residues)
International Agency for Research on Cancer
150 Cours Albert Thomas
69372 Lyon Cedex 08, France

Contact point: J. BAREK

METHOD 10: DESTRUCTION OF CISPLATIN BY REACTION WITH SODIUM DIETHYLDITHIOCARBAMATE

1. SCOPE AND FIELD OF APPLICATION

This method specifies a procedure for the destruction of cisplatin in the following wastes: solid compound (7.1), aqueous solutions, including injectable pharmaceutical preparations (7.2), glassware (7.3) and spills (7.4).

The solution and precipitate produced by this method were tested for mutagenicity using *Salmonella typhimurium* strains TA98, TA100 and TA1535 with and without metabolic activation. No mutagenic activity was detected.

No analytical method was found suitable to verify the degree of destruction; therefore, this method is recommended only on the basis of the absence of mutagenic activity in the residue.

For recommended applications of this procedure, see Methods Index, page 22.

2. REFERENCE

Bannister, S.J., Sternson, L.A. & Repta, A.J. (1979) Urine analysis of platinum species derived from cis-dichlorodiammineplatinum (II) by high-performance liquid chromatography following derivatization with sodium diethyldithiocarbamate. *J. Chromatogr., 173*, 333–342

3. PRINCIPLE

Destruction is effected by decomposition with sodium diethyldithiocarbamate.

4. HAZARDS

4.1 *From cisplatin*

Cisplatin is probably carcinogenic to humans, and appropriate precautions, such as wearing gloves when handling the compound or its solutions, should be taken.

A number of guidelines for the safe handling of antineoplastic agents have been published (Knowles & Virden, 1980; Davis, 1981; Harrison, 1981; Zimmerman *et al.*, 1981; Anderson *et al.*, 1982; National Institutes of Health, 1982; Jones *et al.*, 1983; Solimando, 1983; Stolar *et al.*, 1983; National Study Commission on Cytotoxic Exposure, 1984; American Society of Hospital Pharmacists, 1985).

4.2 *Other hazards*

Sodium hydroxide and its solutions are corrosive and should be handled with care.

In case of skin contact with corrosive chemicals, wash the skin with flowing water for at least 15 min.

Dry sodium nitrate is highly combustible.

5.   REAGENTS

5.1 *For destruction*

Sodium diethyldithiocarbamate	Technical grade
Sodium hydroxide	Technical grade
Sodium hydroxide solution	0.1 mol/L, aqueous (0.4 g/ 100 mL)
Sodium nitrate	Technical grade
Sodium nitrate solution	Saturated, aqueous
Sodium diethyldithiocarbamate solution	0.68 mol/L ($\simeq$ 1 g/100 mL) in 0.1 mol/L sodium hydroxide solution

5.2 *For analysis*

Not applicable.

6.   APPARATUS

Usual laboratory equipment.

7.   PROCEDURE

7.1 *Solid compound*

7.1.1   Estimate the amount of drug to be destroyed.

7.1.2   Dissolve in water.

7.1.3   For every 100 mg cisplatin, add 3 mL sodium diethyldithiocarbamate solution.

7.1.4   Add an equal volume of sodium nitrate solution.

NOTE: A yellow precipitate of the complex of platinum II and diethyldithio-carbamate will form when the platinum concentration is greater than 100 µg/mL.

7.1.5   Discard.

7.2 *Aqueous solutions, including injectable pharmaceutical preparations*

Proceed as in 7.1.

7.3 *Glassware*

Immerse in a 1:1 mixture of sodium diethyldithiocarbamate solution and sodium nitrate solution.

7.4 *Spills*

7.4.1   Isolate the area, and put on suitable protective clothing.

7.4.2   Collect solid, or take up liquid with absorbent material, and place it in a beaker.

7.4.3   Rinse the area with water and take up the rinse on absorbent material. Place the material in the beaker from 7.4.2.

7.4.4   If desired, check the surface for completeness of removal by wiping in with absorbent material moistened with water and analysing the wipe using the method described in Section 7 of Method 9.

7.4.5   Cover the contents of the beaker from 7.4.3 with a 1:1 mixture of sodium diethyldithiocarbamate solution and sodium nitrate solution.

7.4.6   Discard.

8.   ANALYSIS FOR COMPLETENESS OF DEGRADATION

Methods for the analysis of platinum detect the metal ion itself and cannot distinguish between the active starting compound and the inactivated product.

9.   SCHEMATIC REPRESENTATION OF PROCEDURE

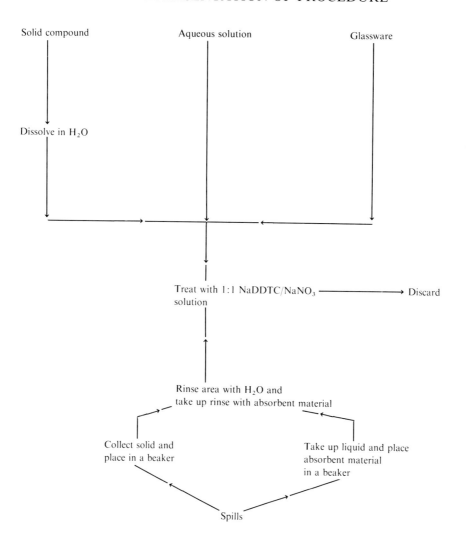

10. ORIGIN OF METHOD

University of Texas System Cancer Center
M.D. Anderson Hospital and Tumor Institute
Departments of Pharmacy and Chemotherapy Research
6723 Bertner Avenue
Houston, Texas 77030, USA

Contact point: J.A. BENVENUTO

METHOD 11: DESTRUCTION OF LOMUSTINE, CHLOROZOTOCIN AND STREPTOZOTOCIN USING HYDROBROMIC ACID IN GLACIAL ACETIC ACID

1. SCOPE AND FIELD OF APPLICATION

This method specifies a procedure for the destruction of lomustine, chlorozotocin and streptozotocin in the following wastes: solid compounds (7.1), solutions in volatile organic solvents (excluding alcohols) (7.2), aqueous solutions (7.3), pharmaceutical preparations (7.4), solutions in methanol or ethanol (7.5), glassware (7.6) and spills of solid compounds or of solutions in volatile organic solvents (including methanol and ethanol) (7.7).

The method has been tested collaboratively using 100 mg solid lomustine, 50 mg solid streptozotocin and a solution of 100 mg chlorozotocin in 4 mL methanol. The method affords better than 98% destruction for the samples tested.

The residues produced by this method were tested for mutagenicity using *Salmonella typhimurium* strains TA1530, TA1535 and TA100 with and without metabolic activation. No mutagenic activity was detected.

NOTE: The method was also tested using PCNU, carmustine and semustine. Destruction of PCNU was not reproducible, and the residues from carmustine and semustine showed mutagenic activity. This method should not be used to destroy PCNU, carmustine or semustine.

For recommended applications of this procedure, see Methods Index, page 22.

2. REFERENCES

Eisenbrand, G. & Preussmann, R. (1970) Eine neue Methode zur kolorimetrischen Bestimmung von Nitrosaminen nach Spaltung der Nitrosogruppe mit Bromwasserstoff in Eisessig. *Arzneimittel. Forsch., 20*, 1513–1517

Johnson, E.M. & Walters, C.L. (1971) The specificity of the release of nitrite from nitrosamines by hydrobromic acid. *Anal. Lett., 4*, 383–386

Lunn, G., Sansone, E.B., Andrews, A.W., Castegnaro, M., Malaveille, C., Michelon, J., Brouet, I. & Keefer, L.K. (1984) *Destruction of carcinogenic and mutagenic N-nitrosamides in laboratory wastes*. In: O'Neill, I.K., von Borstel, R.C., Miller, C.T., Long, J. & Bartsch, H., eds, N-*Nitroso Compounds: Occurrence, Biological Effects and Relevance to Human Cancer (IARC Scientific Publications No. 57)*, Lyon, International Agency for Research on Cancer, pp. 387–398

Preussmann, R. & Eisenbrand, G. (1972) *Problems and recent results in the analytical determination of* N-*nitrosocompounds*. In: *Topics in Chemical Carcinogenesis*, Tokyo, University of Tokyo Press, pp. 323–341

3. PRINCIPLE

In a dry inert solvent, the nitroso group is removed by reaction with a solution of hydrobromic acid in glacial acetic acid; the resulting nitrosyl bromide (NOBr) is removed by flushing with nitrogen to eliminate the possible re-formation of *N*-nitrosoureas.

4. HAZARDS

4.1 *From* N-*nitrosourea drugs*

Some *N*-nitrosoureas are carcinogenic, and gloves must be worn for all operations involving the handling of these compounds or their solutions. Should gloves come into contact with a *N*-nitrosourea solution, they should be changed as quickly as possible to reduce the risk of contact with the skin. The gloves should be discarded after use. Some *N*-nitrosoureas occur as electrostatic powders, and precautions should be taken during the handling of these compounds to avoid their dissemination.

A number of guidelines for the safe handling of antineoplastic agents have been published (Knowles & Virden, 1980; Davis, 1981; Harrison, 1981; Zimmerman *et al.*, 1981; Anderson *et al.*, 1982; National Institutes of Health, 1982; Jones *et al.*, 1983; Solimando, 1983; Stolar *et al.*, 1983; National Study Commission on Cytotoxic Exposure, 1984; American Society of Hospital Pharmacists, 1985).

4.2 *Other hazards*

Sulfuric acid and hydrobromic acid/glacial acetic acid solutions are corrosive and should be handled with care.

In case of skin contact with corrosive chemicals, wash the skin with flowing water for at least 15 min.

5. REAGENTS

5.1 *For destruction*

Hydrobromic acid	30% solution in glacial acetic acid
Glacial acetic acid	Analytical grade
Hydrobromic acid solution	4.5% hydrogen bromide in glacial acetic acid, prepared by diluting the 30% hydrobromic acid/solution 1 to 6 with glacial acetic acid

Ammonium sulfamate	Technical grade
Sodium carbonate	Technical grade
Dichloromethane	Analytical grade (alcohol-free)
Nitrogen gas	
Sulfuric acid (concentrated)	Specific gravity, 1.84; technical grade; $\simeq 18$ mol/L
Sulfuric acid solution	$\simeq 3.6$ mol/L, aqueous

5.2 *For analysis*

Water	Redistilled from glass
Methanol	HPLC grade
Acetonitrile	HPLC grade
Phosphoric acid	Analytical grade
Potassium dihydrogenphosphate (KH_2PO_4)	Analytical grade
KH_2PO_4 solution	0.02 mol/L, aqueous, adjusted to pH 4.8 with phosphoric acid

6. APPARATUS

Usual laboratory equipment and the following items: liquid chromatograph equipped with a reverse-phase ODS column and a UV detection system capable of measurement at 230 nm.

Efficient bubbling system.

7. PROCEDURE

One hundred mg of lomustine dissolved in 2–3 mL dichloromethane or 100 mg solid chlorozotocin or streptozotocin are degraded by 10 mL of a 4.5% solution of hydrobromic acid in glacial acetic acid in 15 min. The nitrosyl bromide formed is removed by flushing with nitrogen for 30 min, to eliminate possible re-formation of *N*-nitrosoureas.

NOTE: The procedure must not be carried out in the presence of water or dimethylsulfoxide.

7.1 *Solid compounds*

7.1.1   Estimate the amount of drug to be destroyed, and calculate the volume of 4.5% hydrobromic acid to be added.

7.1.2   For lomustine, dissolve in dichloromethane.

7.1.3   Add the quantity of 4.5% hydrobromic acid solution calculated in 7.1.1.

NOTE: For lomustine, add at least 10 mL of 4.5% hydrobromic acid solution per 2 mL dichloromethane.

7.1.4   Allow to react at room temperature for about 15 min, then flush out the nitrosyl bromide formed by passing a strong stream of nitrogen through the solution for at least half an hour. Adequate bubbling is essential to avoid re-formation of *N*-nitrosoureas.

NOTE: To avoid contamination of the atmosphere, connect the exhaust of the reaction flask to a flask containing a solution of about 20% ammonium sulfamate in about 3.6 mol/L sulfuric acid.

7.1.5   If desired, check for completeness of destruction using the method described in Section 8.

7.1.6   Dilute with water, and discard.

7.2 *Solutions in volatile organic solvents (excluding alcohols)*

7.2.1   Estimate the amount of drug to be degraded.

7.2.2   Remove solvent by evaporation, using a rotary evaporator under reduced pressure.

7.2.3   Proceed as in 7.1.

7.3 *Aqueous solutions*

NOTE: This method is not appropriate for the treatment of aqueous solutions containing streptozotocin or chlorozotocin. Method 12 must be used for streptozotocin.

7.3.1   Extract with three equal volumes of dichloromethane, each volume of solvent being about equal to the volume of water.

7.3.2   Proceed as in 7.2.

7.4 *Pharmaceutical preparations*

7.4.1   Lomustine (solid compound containing lactose, starch and magnesium stearate): Treat as in 7.1.

7.4.2   Chlorozotocin and streptozotocin (solid compound containing citric acid): Treat as in 7.1.

NOTE: Reconstituted solutions cannot be treated by this method.

7.5 *Solutions in methanol or ethanol*

NOTE: The presence of ethanol or methanol greatly inhibits the rate of denitrosation by hydrobromic acid. Wastes containing methanol or ethanol should, therefore, be collected separately and treated as described below.

7.5.1   Add 4.5% hydrobromic acid solution until the mixture contains less than 15% alcohol and less than 50 mg drug per 40 mL.

7.5.2   Allow to react overnight at room temperature, then remove the nitrosyl bromide formed by flushing with nitrogen for at least 30 min. Adequate bubbling is essential to avoid re-formation of *N*-nitrosoureas.

NOTE: To avoid contamination of the atmosphere, connect the exhaust of the reaction flask to a flask containing a solution of about 20% ammonium sulfamate in about 3.6 mol/L sulfuric acid.

7.5.3   Proceed as in 7.1.5 and 7.1.6.

7.6 *Glassware*

7.6.1   Drain thoroughly and immerse in a 4.5% solution of hydrobromic acid.

7.6.2   Allow to react overnight.

7.6.3   Proceed as in 7.1.5 and 7.1.6.

7.7 *Spills of solid compounds or of solutions in volatile organic solvents (including methanol and ethanol)*

NOTE: This method is not appropriate for the treatment of aqueous spills.

7.7.1   Isolate the area, and put on suitable protective clothing, including breathing apparatus.

7.7.2   For solutions in volatile organic solvents, allow the solvent to evaporate.

7.7.3   Cover the area with an excess of 4.5% solution of hydrobromic acid. Allow to react for at least 1 h.

7.7.4   Add solid sodium carbonate to the treated surface.

7.7.5   To check for completeness of decontamination, wipe the surface with absorbent material moistened with methanol, and analyse the wipe (see Section 8).

8. ANALYSIS FOR COMPLETENESS OF DEGRADATION

Analyse directly by HPLC, using the following conditions:

8.1 *Lomustine*

Column: 25 cm × 3.6 mm i.d., Partisil ODS-2 10 µm

Precolumn: 6.5 cm × 3.6 mm i.d., filled with CO:Pell ODS 30–38 µm

Eluant: Water:methanol:acetonitrile (40:30:30)

Flow rate: 1.5 mL/min

Injection volume: 50 µL

Detector: UV, 230 nm

8.2 *Streptozotocin and chlorozotocin*

Column: 25 cm × 3.6 mm i.d., Partisil ODS-2 10 µm

Precolumn: 6.5 cm × 3.6 mm i.d., filled with CO:Pell ODS 30–38 µm

Eluant: Streptozotocin: 0.02M KH_2PO_4 pH 4.8
        Chlorozotocin: 0.02M KH_2PO_4 pH 4.8:methanol (96:4)

Flow rate: 1.5 mL/min

Injection volume: 50 µL

Detector: UV, 230 nm

9. SCHEMATIC REPRESENTATION OF PROCEDURE

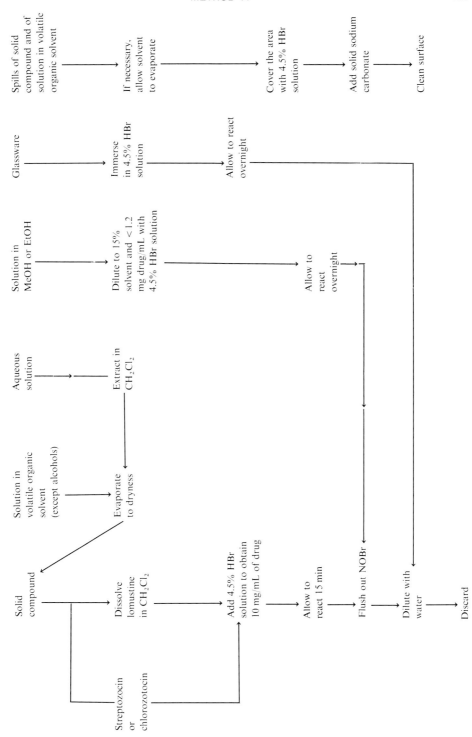

10. ORIGIN OF METHOD

Castegnaro, M., Michelon, J. & Brouet, I.
International Agency for Research on Cancer
150 Cours Albert Thomas
69372 Lyon Cedex 08, France

Contact point: M. CASTEGNARO

Sansone, E.B.
NCI-Frederick Cancer Research Facility
P.O. Box B
Frederick, MD 21701, USA

Contact point: E.B. SANSONE

METHOD 12: DESTRUCTION OF STREPTOZOTOCIN USING POTASSIUM PERMANGANATE/SULFURIC ACID

1. SCOPE AND FIELD OF APPLICATION

This method specifies a procedure for the destruction of streptozotocin in the following wastes: solid compound (6.1), aqueous solutions (6.2), solutions in dimethylformamide (DMF) or dimethylsulfoxide (DMSO) (6.3), solutions in volatile organic solvents (6.4), pharmaceutical solutions (6.5), glassware (6.6) and spills (6.7).

The method has been tested collaboratively using 40 mg streptozotocin in aqueous solution; it affords better than 99.5% destruction.

The residues produced by this method were tested for mutagenicity using *Salmonella typhimurium* strains TA1530, TA1535 and TA100 with and without metabolic activation. No mutagenic activity was detected.

> NOTE: This method was also tested for lomustine, carmustine, semustine, PCNU and chlorozotocin. Although chemical destruction of the drugs was satisfactory, the residues showed high mutagenic activity. The method should not be used to destroy these compounds.

For recommended applications of this method, see Methods Index, page 22.

2. PRINCIPLE

Destruction is effected by oxidation with a solution of potassium permanganate in sulfuric acid.

3. HAZARDS

3.1 *From streptozotocin*

Streptozotocin is carcinogenic to some animal species, and gloves must be worn for all operations involving the handling of this compound or its solutions. Should gloves come into contact with a streptozotocin solution, they should be changed as quickly as possible to reduce the risk of contact with the skin. The gloves should be discarded after use. Some *N*-nitrosoureas occur as electrostatic powders, and precautions should be taken during the handling of these compounds to avoid their dissemination.

A number of guidelines for the safe handling of antineoplastic agents have been published (Knowles & Virden, 1980; Davis, 1981; Harrison, 1981; Zimmerman *et al.*, 1981; Anderson *et al.*, 1982; National Institutes of Health, 1982; Jones *et al.*, 1983; Solimando, 1983; Stolar *et al.*,1983; National Study Commission on Cytotoxic Exposure, 1984; American Society of Hospital Pharmacists, 1985).

3.2 *Other hazards*

Concentrated sulfuric acid and sodium hydroxide are corrosive and should be handled with care.

Care should be taken in the preparation of solutions of potassium permanganate in sulfuric acid; never add solid potassium permanganate to concentrated sulfuric acid.

The dilution of concentrated sulfuric acid with water is an extremely exothermic reaction; always add the acid to the water, never the reverse, and remove heat by cooling in a cold-water bath.

Potassium permanganate is a strong oxidizing agent; care must be taken not to mix it with concentrated reducing agents.

In case of skin contact with corrosive chemicals, wash the skin with flowing water for at least 15 min.

4.   REAGENTS

4.1 *For destruction*

Potassium permanganate	Technical grade
Sulfuric acid (concentrated)	Specific gravity, 1.84 (about 18 mol/L); technical grade
Sulfuric acid solution	$\simeq 3$ mol/L, aqueous (see 3.2, Hazards)
Potassium permanganate/sulfuric acid solution	To 100 mL of a 3 mol/L sulfuric acid solution, add 4.7 g solid potassium permanganate

NOTE: The reagent should always be freshly prepared on the day of use.

Ascorbic acid or sodium bisulfite	Technical grade
Ascorbic acid or sodium bisulfite solution	$\simeq 50$ g/L, aqueous
Sodium hydroxide	Technical grade
Sodium hydroxide solution	$\simeq 2$ mol/L, aqueous ($\simeq 8$ g/100 mL)
Sodium carbonate	Technical grade

4.2 *For analysis*

Ascorbic acid	Analytical grade
Water	Redistilled from glass
Potassium dihydrogenphosphate (KH_2PO_4)	Analytical grade
Phosphoric acid	Analytical grade
KH_2PO_4 solution	0.02 mol/L, aqueous; adjusted to pH 4.8 with phosphoric acid

5. APPARATUS

Usual laboratory equipment and the following items: liquid chromatograph equipped with a reverse-phase ODS column and a UV detection system capable of measurement at 230 nm.

6. PROCEDURE

Forty-eight mg of streptozotocin dissolved in 10 mL of 3 mol/L sulfuric acid are destroyed by 2 g potassium permanganate in 10–12 h.

6.1 *Solid compound*

6.1.1   For each 48 mg of drug, add 10 mL of 3 mol/L sulfuric acid.

6.1.2   Place flask on a magnetic stirrer; add 2 g potassium permanganate per 10 mL of solution from 6.1.1.

6.1.3   Stir overnight.

6.1.4   If desired, check for completeness of destruction using the method described in Section 7.

6.1.5   Neutralize with 8 g/100 mL sodium hydroxide solution and discard.

6.2 *Aqueous solutions*

6.2.1   If necessary, dilute with water to obtain a maximum content of $\simeq$ 5 mg/ mL of drug.

6.2.2   Add slowly, with stirring, enough concentrated sulfuric acid to obtain a 3 mol/L solution and allow to cool to room temperature (see 3.2, Hazards).

6.2.3   Proceed as in 6.1.2 to 6.1.5.

6.3 *Solutions in DMF or DMSO*

6.3.1   Dilute with water to obtain a maximum concentration of 15% solvent and not more than 5 mg/mL streptozotocin.

6.3.2   Proceed as in 6.2.2 and 6.2.3.

6.4 *Solutions in volatile organic solvents*

6.4.1   Remove the solvent by evaporation, using a rotary evaporator under reduced pressure.

6.4.2   Proceed as in 6.1.

6.5 *Pharmaceutical solutions*

Solid compound containing citric acid diluted with saline (10 mg/ml) or 5% dextrose (0.1 mg/ml): proceed as in 6.2.

NOTE: To avoid frothing in solutions containing dextrose, add potassium permanganate in small increments.

6.6 *Glassware*

6.6.1   Immerse in a freshly prepared solution of potassium permanganate/sulfuric acid. Allow to react 10–12 h.

6.6.2   Clean the glass by immersion in a solution of ascorbic acid or sodium bisulfite.

6.7 *Spills*

6.7.1   Isolate the area, and put on suitable protective clothing.

6.7.2   Collect the solid, or take up the liquid on absorbent material, and place the material in a beaker under a well-ventilated fume hood.

6.7.3   Rinse the area with water. Take up the rinse with absorbent material, and place the material in the beaker from 6.7.2.

6.7.4   If desired, check the surface for completeness of removal by wiping it with absorbent material moistened with water and analysing the wipe (see Section 7).

6.7.5   Cover the contents of the beaker from 6.7.3 with potassium permanganate/sulfuric acid solution and allow to react overnight.

6.7.6   Neutralize with 8 g/100 mL sodium hydroxide solution. Discard.

7.   ANALYSIS FOR COMPLETENESS OF DEGRADATION

7.1 Add ascorbic until the solution becomes colourless.

7.2 Analyse by HPLC, using the following conditions or any other suitable system:

Column: 25 cm × 3.6 mm i.d., Partisil ODS-2 10 μm

Pre-column: 6.5 cm × 3.6 mm i.d., filled with CO:Pell ODS 30–38 μm

Eluant: 0.02 mol/L KH_2PO_4, pH 4.8

Flow rate: 1.5 mL/min

Injection volume: 50 μL

Detector: UV, 230 nm

8.   SCHEMATIC REPRESENTATION OF PROCEDURE

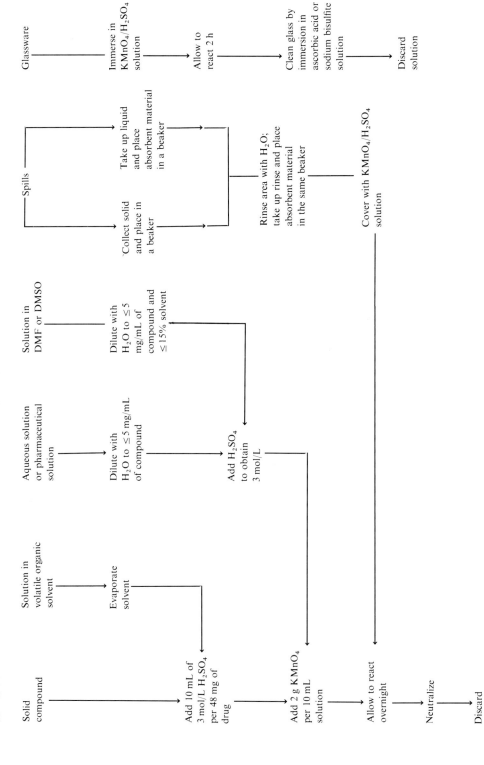

9.   ORIGIN OF METHOD
     Castegnaro, M., Brouet, I. & Michelon, J.
     International Agency for Research on Cancer
     150 Cours Albert Thomas
     69372 Lyon Cedex 08, France

     Contact point: M. CASTEGNARO

APPENDIX A
NOMENCLATURE AND CHEMICAL AND PHYSICAL DATA
ON THE ANTINEOPLASTIC AGENTS CONSIDERED

1. **Doxorubicin**

   Nomenclature

   Chemical Abstracts Services Registry Number: 23214-92-8

   Chemical Abstracts Name: (8S-*cis*)-10-[(3-Amino-2,3,6-trideoxy-α-L-lyxohexa-pyranosyl)oxy]-7,8,9,10-tetrahydro-6,8,11-trihydroxy-8-(hydroxyacetyl)-1-methoxy-5,12-naphthacenedione

   Synonyms: Adriablastin; adriablastina; adriamycin; 10-[(3-amino-2,3,6-trideoxy-D-lyxohexopyranosyl)oxy]-8-glycosyl-7,8,9,10-tetrahydro-6,8,11-trihydroxy-1-methoxy-5,12-naphthacenedione; 1,2,3,4,6,11-hexahydro-4β,-5,12-trihydroxy-4-(hydroxyacetyl)-10-methoxy-6,11-dioxonaphthacene-1β-yl-3-amino-2,3,6-trideoxy-α-L-lyxohexopyranoside; 14-hydroxydaunomycin; 14′-hydroxy-daunomycin; FI 106; NSC-123127

   Molecular and structural information

   Molecular formula: $C_{27}H_{29}NO_{11}$

   Molecular weight: 543.54

   Structural formula:

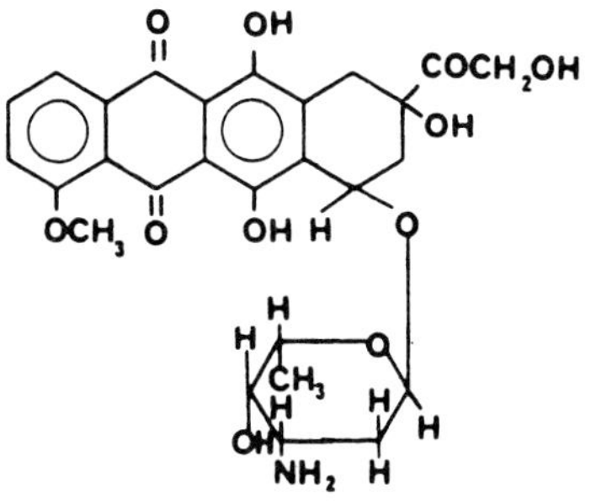

   Physical properties

   Data obtained from Wade (1977), Vigevani & Williamson (1980) or Windholz (1983), unless otherwise specified

   Description: Orange-red, thin needles; reddish powder

Melting-point: 204–205 °C (with decomposition); 205 °C (decomposes) (Arca-
                    mone *et al.*, 1975)

Optical rota- $[\alpha]_D^{20} + 248°$ (C = 0.1 in methanol) (Arcamone *et al.*, 1969);
tion: $[\alpha]_D^{25} + 255°$ (C = 0.1 in methanol)

Solubility: Soluble in water, methanol and aqueous ethanol. Practically
                    insoluble in acetone, benzene, chloroform, ethylether and
                    petroleum ether
                    Aqueous solutions are yellow orange at acid pHs and violet
                    blue at pHs above 9

Stability: Aqueous solutions are stable at pH 3 to 6.5, but decompose
                    as the pH increases in the range 6.5 to 12 (Vigevani & William-
                    son, 1980)
                    Aqueous solutions are unchanged after 1 month at 5 °C but
                    unstable at higher temperatures (Windholz, 1983)

Spectral data: UV λ_{max} (E_1^1) in methanol: 233 (658), 253 (440), 290 (145), 477
                    (225), 495 (223), 529 (124) (Arcamone *et al.*, 1969)
                    UV and NMR spectra are described by Smith *et al.* (1977) and
                    Vigevani & Williamson (1980)
                    IR spectra are described by Arcamone *et al.* (1969) and Vigeva-
                    ni & Williamson (1980)
                    Mass spectra are given by Vigevani & Williamson (1980).

2.   **Daunorubicin**

Nomenclature

Chemical Abstracts Services Registry Number: 20830-81-3

Chemical Abstracts Name: (8S-*cis*)-8-Acetyl-10-[(3-amino-2,3,6-trideoxy-α-L-
lyxohexapyranosy)oxy]-7,8,9,10-tetrahydro-6,8,11-tetrahydroxy-1-methoxy-
5,12-naphthacenedione

Synonyms: Acetyladriamycin; 8-acetyl-10-[(3-amino-2,3,6-trideoxy-α-L-lyxo-
hexapyranosyl)oxy]-7,8,9,10-tetrahydro-6,8,11-trihydroxy-1-methoxy-(8S, 10S)-
5,12-naphthacenedione; 3-acetyl-1,2,3,4,6,11-hexahydro-3,5,12-trihydroxy-10-
methoxy-6,11-dioxo-1-naphthacenyl-3-amino-2,3,6-trideoxy-α-L-lyxohexapyra-
noside (1S 3S); cerubidin; daunomycin; daunorubicine; leukaemomycin C; NSC
82151; RP 13057; rubidomycin; rubomycin C; rubomycin C_1

Molecular and structural information

Molecular formula: $C_{27}H_{29}NO_{10}$

Molecular weight: 527.5

Structural formula:

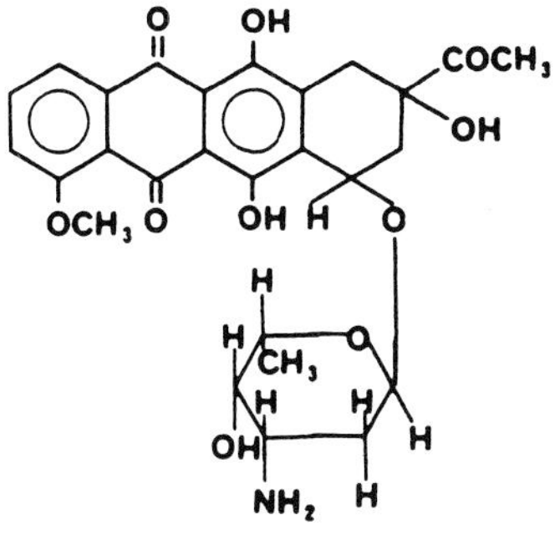

Physical properties

Data obtained from Wade (1977) or Windholz (1983)

Description:	Thin red needles; orange-red hygroscopic microcrystalline powder
Melting-point:	188–190 °C (with decomposition)
Optical rotation:	$[\alpha]_D^{20} + 248 \pm 5°$ (C = 0.05–0.1 in methanol)
Solubility:	Soluble in water, methanol and aqueous alcohols Practically insoluble in chloroform, ether and benzene The colour of aqueous solutions changes from pink at acid pH to blue at alkaline pH
Spectral data:	UV λ_{max} (E$_1^1$) in methanol: 234 (665), 252 (462), 290 (153), 480 (214), 495 (218), 532 (112).

3. Methotrexate

Nomenclature

Chemical Abstracts Services Registry Number: 59-05-2

Chemical Abstracts Name: L-Glutamic acid, *N*-(4-{[(2,4-diamino-6-pteridinyl)-methyl]methylamino}benzoyl-

Synonyms: A-methopterin; amethopterin; amethopterine; 4-amino-4-deoxy-N^{10}-methylpteroylglutamic acid; 4-amino-10-methylfolic acid; 4-amino-N^{10}-methylpteroylglutamic acid; antifulan; *N*-bismethylpteroylglutamic acid; CL-14377; *N*-{*para*[(2-4-diaminopteridin-6-yl-methyl)methylamino]benzoyl}-L-glutamic acid; *N*-(*p*{[(2,4-diamino-6-pteridinyl)methyl]methylamino}benzoyl-,L-; EMT 25,299; glutamic acid; glutamic acid, *N*-(*p*{[(2,4-diamino-6-pteridinyl)methyl]-methylamino}benzoyl)-,L-(+)-8 CI; HDMTX; ledertrexate; α-methopterin; methotrexate specia; methotrexatum; methylaminopterin; MEXATE; MTX; NCI-CO4671; NSC 740; R 9985

Molecular and structural information

Molecular formula: $C_{20}H_{22}N_8O_5$

Molecular weight: 454.4

Structural formula:

Physical properties

Data obtained from Wade (1977) or Windholz (1983), unless otherwise specified

Description:	Bright yellow-orange, odourless crystalline powder (Chamberlin *et al.*, 1976) containing not less than 85% 4-amino-10-methylfolic acid
Melting-point:	Decomposes at 185–204 °C (monohydrate)
Optical rotation:	$[\alpha]^{21}_{589} = 20.4 \pm 0.6°$ (C = 1; 0.1 N NaOH) (Chamberlin *et al.*, 1976)
Solubility:	Practically insoluble in water, ethanol, chloroform and diethyl-ether; freely soluble in dilute solutions of alkaline hydroxides or carbonates; soluble in dilute hydrochloric acid For medical use, solutions are prepared as follows: 10 mg/mL 0.9% NaCl; 5% dextrose, pH 7.0–8.8; 50 mg/mL sterile water, pH 7.0–8.8 (National Cancer Institute, 1983)
Stability:	Sensitive to hydrolysis, oxidation and light. Bottles of tablets are stable for at least three years at room temperature (20–25 °C) Medical solutions described above are stable for at least one week at room temperature (National Cancer Institute, 1983)

Spectral data: UV λ_{max} (A_1^1) in 0.0IN HCl: 243 (388), 307 (475); in 0.IN NaOH: 258 (544), 303 (546), 372 (177)
IR and NMR spectra have been tabulated (Chamberlin *et al.*, 1976)
Field desorption mass spectra are available (Przybylski *et al.*, 1982).

4. Dichloromethotrexate

Nomenclature

Chemical Abstracts Services Registry Number: 528-74-5

Chemical Abstracts Names: L-Glutamic acid, *N*-(3,5-dichloro-4-{[(2,4-diamino-6-pteridinyl)methyl]methylamino}benzoyl)-; glutamic acid, *N*-(3,5-dichloro-4-{[(2,4-diamino-6-pteridinyl)methyl]methylamino}benzoyl)-, L-

Synonyms: 4-Amino-10-methyl-3',5'-dichloro-pteroyl glutamic acid; 3',5'-dichloroamethopterin; 3',5'-dichloromethotrexate; methotrexate, dichloro-; NSC 29630

Molecular and structural information

Molecular formula: $C_{20}H_{20}Cl_2N_8O_5$

Molecular weight: 523.4

Structural formula:

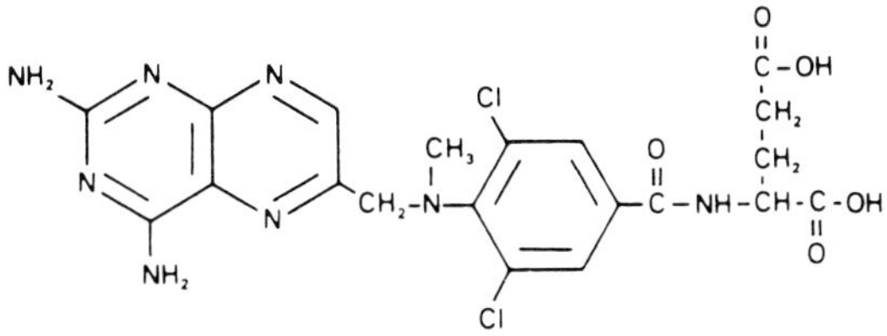

Physical properties

Data obtained from Chamberlin *et al.* (1976) and Windholz (1983)

Description: Square platelets from 50% aqueous alcohol; bright-yellow odourless crystalline powder

Melting-point: 185–204 °C (monohydrate)

Optical rota- $[\alpha]_{589}^{21} = 20.4 \pm 0.6°$ (C = 1; 0.1 N NaOH)
tion:

Solubility: Practically insoluble in water, ethanol, chloroform and diethyl-
                   ether; freely soluble in dilute solutions of alkaline hydroxides
                   and carbonates; soluble in dilute hydrochloric acid

Spectral data: UV λ_{max} (A_1^1) in 0.1 N NaOH: 258 (488), 370 (145); in 0.1 N
                   HCl: 240 (442), 330 (231)
                   IR and NMR spectra are available.

5. **Cyclophosphamide**

Nomenclature

Chemical Abstracts Services Registry Number: 6055-19-2 or 50-18-0 (anhydrous form)

Chemical Abstracts Name: $2H$-1,3,2-Oxazaphosphorin-2-amine, N,N-bis(2-chloroethyl)tetrahydro-, 2-oxide monohydrate

Synonyms: 2-[Bis(2-chloroethyl)amino]-1-oxa-3-aza-2-phosphocyclohexane 2-oxide monohydrate; 1-bis(2-chloroethyl)amino-1-oxo-2-aza-5-oxaphosphoridine monohydrate; 2-[bis(2-chloroethyl)amino]tetrahydro-2H-1,3,2-oxazaphosphorine 2-oxide monohydrate; 2-[bis(2-chloroethyl)amino]tetrahydro[2H]-1,3,2-oxazaphosphorine 2-oxide monohydrate; [bis(chloro-2-ethyl)-amino]-2-tetrahydro-3,4,5,6-oxazaphosphorine-1,3,2-oxide-2 monohydrate; N,N-bis(2-chloroethyl)-N'-(3-hydroxypropyl)phosphorodiamidic acid intramolecular ester monohydrate; bis(2-chloroethyl)phosphoramide cyclic propanolamide ester monohydrate; N,N-bis(β-chloroethyl)-N',O-propylenephosphoric acid ester amide monohydrate; N,N-bis(β-chloroethyl)-N,O-trimethylene-phosphoric acid ester diamide monohydrate; B 518; CB-4564; clafen; cyclic N',O-propylene ester of N,N-bis(2-chloroethyl)phosphoro-diamidic acid monohydrate; cyclophosphamid; cyclophosphamidum; cyclophosphan; cyclophosphane; cyclophosphanum; cytophosphan; cytoxan; 2-[di(2-chloroethyl)amino]-1-oxa-3-aza-2-phosphacyclohexane-2-oxide monohydrate; N,N-di(2-chloroethyl)amino-N,O-propylene phosphoric acid ester diamide monohydrate; endoxan; endoxana; endoxan-asta; endoxan R; enduxan; genoxal; mitoxan; NSC-26271; procytox; semdoxan; sendoxan; senduxan

Molecular and structural information

Molecular formula: $C_7H_{15}Cl_2N_2O_2P.H_2O$

Molecular weight: 279.1

Structural formula:
* 2 optical isomers

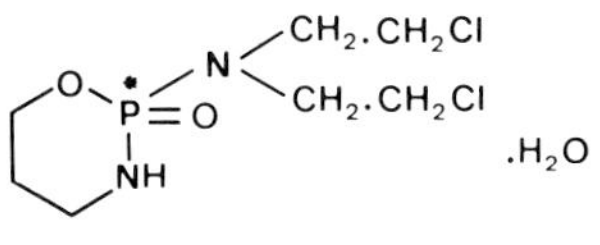

Physical properties

Data obtained from Wade (1977) or Windholz (1983), unless otherwise specified

Description:	Fine white, odourless or almost odourless crystalline powder with a slightly bitter taste
Melting-point:	41–45 °C (monohydrate); 49.5–53 °C
Solubility:	Soluble in water (40 g/L) and ethanol (1 to 1); slightly soluble in benzene, ethylene glycol, carbon tetrachloride, dioxane; sparingly soluble in ether and acetone
Stability:	Sensitive to oxidation, moisture and light; liquifies upon loss of its water of crystallization
Spectral data:	NMR spectra are available (Zon *et al.*, 1977).

6. **Ifosfamide**

Nomenclature

Chemical Abstracts Services Registry Number: 3778-73-2

Chemical Abstracts Name: 2*H*-1,3,2-Oxazaphosphorine-2-amine,*N*,3-bis(2-chloroethyl)tetrahydro-, 2-oxide

Synonyms: A 4942; asta Z 4942; 3-(2-chloroethyl)-2-[(2-chloroethyl)amino]perhydro-2*H*-1,3,2-oxazaphosphorine 2-oxide; 3-(2-chloroethyl)-2-[(2-chloroethyl)amino]tetrahydro-2*H*-1,3,2-oxazaphosphorine 2 oxide; cyfos; holoxan 1000; ifosfamid; iphosphamid; iphosphamide; isoendoxan; isofosfamide; isofosfamidum; isophosphamide; mitoxena; MJF 9325; naxamide; NSC 109724; Z 4942

Molecular and structural information

Molecular formula: $C_7H_{15}Cl_2N_2O_2P$

Molecular weight: 261.1

Structural formula:
* 2 optical isomers

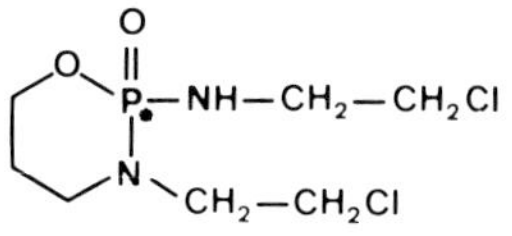

Physical properties

Data obtained from Handelsman *et al.* (1974), unless otherwise specified

Description:	Crystals from anhydrous ether (Windholz, 1983); white crystals
Melting-point:	39–41 °C (Windholz, 1983); 48–50 °C; 50–55 °C (Zon *et al.*, 1977)
Solubility:	Soluble in water (1 in 10) and carbon disulfide (1.5 in 100); very soluble in dichloromethane For medical use, solutions are prepared in sterile water (50 or 100 mg/mL), to pH 4–7 (National Cancer Institute, 1983)
Stability:	Sensitive to hydrolysis, oxidation and heat Reconstituted solutions for medical use are stable for at least seven days (National Cancer Institute, 1983)
Spectral data:	IR and NMR spectra are available (Handelsman *et al.*, 1974; Zon *et al.*, 1977).

7. Vincristine sulfate

Nomenclature

Chemical Abstracts Services Registry Number: 2068-78-2

Chemical Abstracts Name: Vincaleukoblastine, 22-oxo-, sulfate (1:1) (salt)

Synonyms: 37231; DES-N_a-methyl-N_a-formylvinblastine sulfate; kyocristine; LCR; LCR sulfate; leurocristine sulfate; leurocristine, sulfate (1:1) (salt); NSC 67574; oncovin; onkovin; 22-oxovincaleukoblastine; VCR; VCR sulfate; vincrisul

Molecular and structural information

Molecular formula: $C_{46}H_{56}N_4O_{10} \cdot H_2SO_4$

Molecular weight: 923.0

Structural formula:

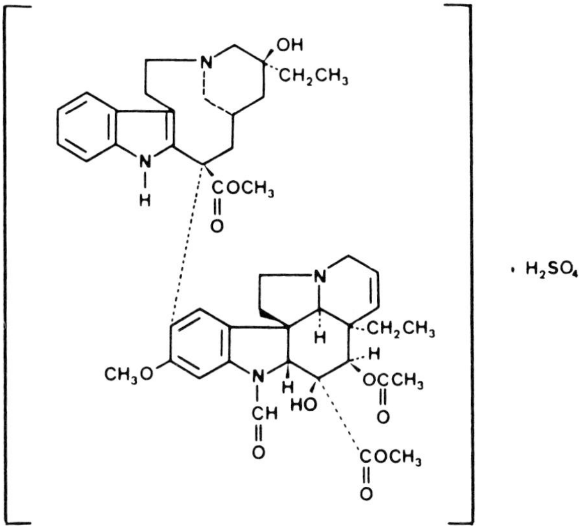

Physical properties

Data obtained from Wade (1977) or Burns (1972)

Description:	White to slightly yellow, odourless, very hygroscopic, amorphous or crystalline powder
Melting-point:	After recrystallization from absolute ethanol, 273–281 °C
Optical rotation:	$[\alpha]_D^{25}$ 8.5 (C = 0.8 in methanol)
Solubility:	Soluble in water (1 in 2), ethanol (1 in 600), chloroform (1 in 30) and methanol; insoluble in diethylether
Stability:	Sensitive to hydrolysis, oxidation and heat
Spectral data:	UV λ_{max} (E_1^1) in 95% ethanol: 221 (510), 255 (167), 296 (169) IR and NMR spectra have been tabulated (Burns, 1972).

8. Vinblastine sulfate

Nomenclature

Chemical Abstracts Services Registry Number: 143-67-9

Chemical Abstracts Name: Vincaleukoblastine, sulfate (1:1) (salt)

Synonyms: Exal; 1*H*-indolizino(8,1-*cd*)carbazole, vincaleukoblastine deriv.; 29060-LE; 2*H*-3,7-methanoazacycloundecino(5,4-*b*)indole, vincaleukoblastine deriv.; NSC 49842; velban; velbe; vincaleucoblastine sulfate; vincaleukoblastine sulfate; VLB sulfate

Molecular and structural information

Molecular formula: $C_{46}H_{58}N_4O_9 \cdot H_2SO_4$

Molecular weight: 909.1

Structural formula:

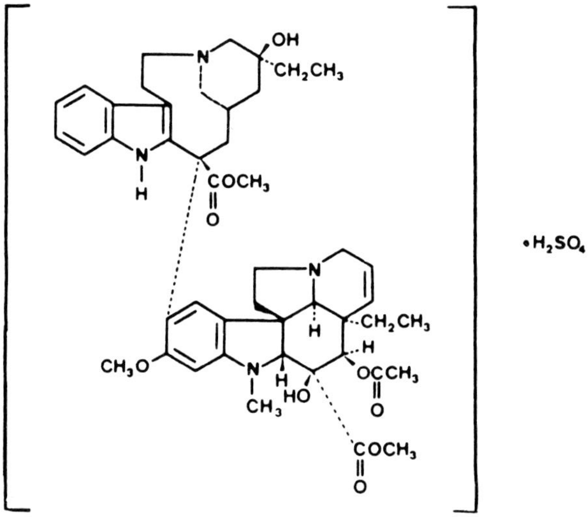

Physical properties

Data obtained from Wade (1977), Windholz (1983) or Burns (1972)

Description:	White to slightly yellow, odourless, hygroscopic, amorphous or crystalline powder. Loses more than 17% of its weight on drying
Melting-point:	284–285 °C with decomposition (monohydrate)
Optical rotation:	$[\alpha]_D^{26}$ –28° (C = 1.01 in methanol)
Solubility:	Soluble in water (1 in 10), ethanol (1 in 12 200), chloroform (1 in 50) and methanol; insoluble in diethylether
Stability:	Sensitive to hydrolysis, oxidation and heat

Spectral data: UV λ_{max} (A_1^1) in 95% ethanol: 214 (592), 246 (131), 262 (176), 287 (143), 296 (127) (11 500)
IR and NMR spectra are given by Burns (1972).

9. 6-Thioguanine

Nomenclature

Chemical Abstracts Services Registry Number: 154-42-7

Chemical Abstracts Name: 6*H*-Purine-6-thione, 2-amino-1,7-dihydro-

Synonyms: 2-Amino-6-mercaptopurine hemihydrate; purine-6-thiol, 2-amino; 6-thioguanine; 6-TG

Molecular and structural information

Molecular formula: $C_5H_5N_5S$

Molecular weight: 167.2

Structural formula:

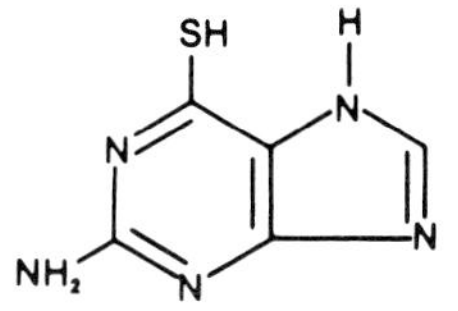

Physical properties

Description: Needles from water; pale-yellow odourless, or almost odourless, crystalline powder

Melting-point: $> 360\,^{\circ}C$

Solubility: Insoluble in water, ethanol and chloroform; very soluble in dilute solutions of alkali hydroxides
For medical use, solutions are prepared as 15 mg/ml of 0.9% NaCl adjusted to pH 11–12 with NaOH

10. 6-Mercaptopurine

Nomenclature
Chemical Abstracts Services Registry Number: 50-42-2

Chemical Abstracts Name: 6*H*-Purine-6-thione, 1,7-dihydro-

Synonyms: Hypoxantine, thio-; IDN 1226; ismipur; leukerin; leupurin; mercaleukin; 6-mercaptopurin; mercaptopurine; mercaptopurinol; 7-mercapto-1,3,4,6-tetrazaindene; mercapurin; MERN; 6MP; NCI-C04886; NSC 755; purine 6-mercapto; 1H-purine, 6-mercapto; purinethiol; purine-6-thiol (8CI); 6-purinethiol; 3H-purine-6-thiol; purinethol; thiohypoxanthine; 6-thiopurine; 6-thioxopurine

Molecular and structural information
Molecular formula: $C_5H_4N_4S$

Molecular weight: 152.2

Structural formula:

Physical properties
Data obtained from Wade (1977), Weast (1977) or Windholz (1983), unless otherwise specified

Description:	Monohydrate, yellow prisms from water; yellow, odourless, almost tasteless crystalline powder
Melting-point:	313–314 °C (decomposition)
Solubility:	Almost insoluble in water, acetone, chloroform and ether; soluble 1 in 950 in ethanol; soluble in solutions of alkali hydroxide and in dilute sulfuric acid; soluble in boiling water (1 in 100) For medical use, solutions are prepared as 10 mg of sodium salt per mL of sterile water, pH 10–11 (National Cancer Institute, 1983)
Stability:	Sensitive to oxidation and light; becomes anhydrous at 140 °C
Spectral data:	UV λ_{max} (A_1^1) in 0.1 N NaOH: 230 (919), 312 (1288); in 0.1 N HCl: 222 (607), 327 (1400); in methanol: 216 (587), 329 (1268).

11. Cisplatin

Nomenclature
Chemical Abstracts Services Registry Number: 15663-27-1

Chemical Abstracts Name: Platinum, diammine dichloro-, (SP-4-2)-

Synonyms: CACP; CDDP; CPDC; DDP; *cis*-DDP; *cis*-diaminodichloroplatinum; *cis*-diaminodichloroplatinum (II); *cis*-diamminedichloroplatinum; *cis*-diamminedichloroplatinum (II); *cis*-diammineplatinum (II) chloride; *cis*-dichlorodiaminoplatinum; *cis*-dichlorodiaminoplatinum (II); *cis*-dichlorodiammineplatinum; *cis*-dichlorodiammineplatinum (II); neoplatin; NSC 119875; PDD; platinex; platinol; *cis*-platinous diaminodichloride; *cis*-platinum; *cis*-platinum (II); *cis*-platinum diaminodichloride; *cis*-platinum (II) diaminodichloride; platinum diamminedichloride; *cis*-platinum diamminedichloride; *cis*-platinum (II) diamminedichloride; *cis*-platyl

Molecular and structural information
Molecular formula: $Cl_2H_6N_2Pt$

Molecular weight: 300.05

Structural formula:

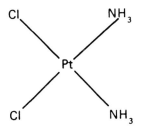

Physical properties
Data obtained from Windholz (1983) and Kauffman & Cowan (1963), unless otherwise specified

Description: Deep-yellow solid

Melting-point: 270° (decomposition)

Solubility: Slightly soluble in water (0.253/100) at 25 °C; insoluble in most common organic solvents, except dimethylformamide

Stability: Slowly changes to the *trans* form in aqueous solutions.
Intact vials are stable for at least four years at 2–8 °C and two years at ambient temperature (22–25 °C)
Interacts with aluminium components of needles, syringes and catheters, forming a black precipitate.

12. Streptozotocin

Nomenclature
Chemical Abstracts Services Registry Number: 18883-66-4

Chemical Abstracts Name: D-Glucose, 2-deoxy-2-{[(methylnitrosamino)car-bonyl]amino}-

Synonyms: 2-Deoxy-2-{[(methylnitrosamino)carbonyl]amino}-D-glucopyranose; 2-deoxy-2-(3-methyl-3-nitrosoureido)-D-glucopyranose; glucopyranose, 2-de-oxy-2-(3-methyl-3-nitrosoureido)-,D-; *N*-d-glucosyl(2)-*N'*-nitrosomethylharn-stoff; *N*-D-glucosyl-(2)-*N'*-nitrosomethylurea; NCI-CO 3167; NSC 37915 (Wade, 1977); NSC 85998; STR; streptozocin; STZ; U-9889; zanosar

Molecular and structural information

Molecular formula: $C_8H_{15}N_3O_7$

Molecular weight: 265.2

Structural formula:

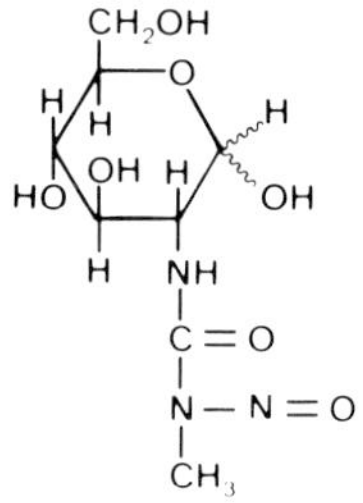

Physical properties

Data obtained from Windholz (1983), unless otherwise specified

Description:	Pointed platelets or prisms from 95% ethanol
Melting-point:	115 °C (decomposition) (White, 1963)
Optical rotation:	Streptozotocin is a mixture of α and β stereoisomers; $[\alpha]_D^{25}$ varies widely between $+15°$ and $+68°$; aqueous solutions rapidly undergo mutarotation to an equilibrium value of $[\alpha]_D^{25}$ $+39°$ (Herr *et al.*, 1967; Rudas, 1972)
Solubility:	Soluble in water, lower alcohols and ketones; insoluble in non-polar organic solvents
Stability:	Decomposes to diazomethane in alkaline solutions at 0 °C (Herr *et al.*, 1967)
Spectral data:	UV λ_{max} in ethanol: 228 nm, $E_1^1 = 240$ (Herr *et al.*, 1967); 380, 394, 412 nm (Rudas, 1972)

13. **Chlorozotocin**

Nomenclature

Chemical Abstracts Services Registry Number: 54749-90-5

Chemical Abstracts Name: D-Glucose, 2-({[(2-chloroethyl)nitrosamino]carbonyl}amino)-2-deoxy-

Synonyms: 2({[(2-Chloroethyl)nitrosamino]carbonyl}amino)-2-deoxy-;   1-(2-chloroethyl)-1-nitroso-3-(D-glucos-2-yl)urea;   2-[3-(2-chloroethyl)-3-nitroso-ureido]-2-deoxy-D′-glucopyranose; DCNU; D-glucopyranose; NSC 178248; NSC 178,248

Molecular and structural information

Molecular formula: $C_9H_{16}ClN_3O_7$

Molecular weight: 313.7

Structural formula:

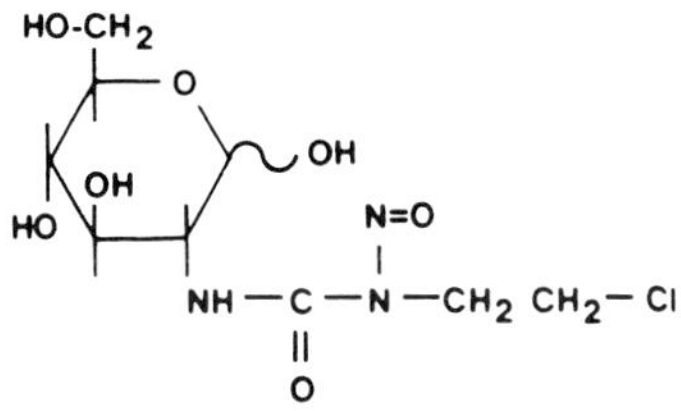

Physical properties

Data obtained from Windholz (1983), unless otherwise specified

Description:	Ivory-coloured crystals; light-yellow crystals (Johnston *et al.*, 1979)
Melting-point:	147–148 °C (decomposition with evolution of gas); 140–141 °C (decomposition) (Johnston *et al.*, 1975)
Optical rotation:	$[\alpha]_D^{25}$: $-53°$ (0 h) (C 1.0, H_2O); $-36°$ (2.5 h); $-19°$ (20 h) (Johnston *et al.*, 1979)
Spectral data:	IR and PMR spectra are available (Johnston *et al.*, 1975).

14. Lomustine

Nomenclature

Chemical Abstracts Services Registry Number: 13010-47-4

Chemical Abstracts Name: Urea, *N*-(2-chloroethyl)-*N'*-cyclohexyl-*N*-nitroso-

Synonyms: Belustine; CeCeNU; Cee NU; chloroethylcyclohexylnitrosourea; 1-(2-chloroethyl)-3-cyclohexyl-1-nitrosourea; 1-(2-chloroethyl)-3-cyclohexyl-nitrosourea; CCNU; ICIG 1109; NSC 79037; RB 1509

Molecular and structural information
Molecular formula: $C_9H_{16}ClN_3O_2$

Molecular weight: 233.7

Structural formula:

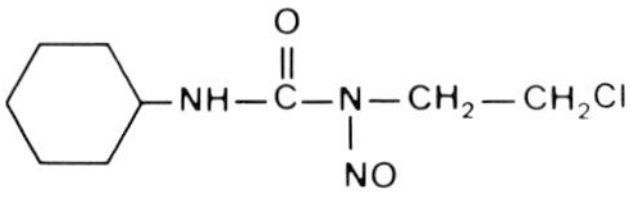

$$\text{cyclohexyl}-NH-\overset{\overset{\displaystyle O}{\|}}{C}-\underset{\underset{\displaystyle NO}{|}}{N}-CH_2-CH_2Cl$$

Physical properties
Data obtained from Windholz (1983) or Baker (1980), unless otherwise specified

Description: Yellow powder

Melting-point: $90\,°C$

Solubility: <0.05 mg/mL in water, 0.1 N sodium hydroxide, 0.1 N hy-drochloric acid or 10% ethanol; 70 mg/mL in absolute ethanol

Stability: Sensitive to oxidation and hydrolysis; forms alkylating and carbamoylating intermediates. Half-life of 117 min at $25\,°C$ and neutral pH (Schein *et al.*, 1978)

Spectral data: Infrared and nuclear magnetic resonance spectra have been reported (Lown & Chauhan, 1981b).

15. Carmustine

Nomenclature

Chemical Abstracts Services Registry Number: 154-93-8

Chemical Abstracts Name: Urea, N,N'-bis(2-chloroethyl)-N-nitroso-

Synonyms: BCNU; BiCNU; 1,3-bis(2-chloroethyl)-1-nitrosourea; 1,3-bis(2-chloroethyl)nitrosourea; bis(2-chloroethyl)nitrosourea; 1,3-bis(β-chloroethyl)-1-nitrosourea; N,N'-bis(2-chloroethyl)-N-nitrosourea; 1,3-di-(2-chloroethyl)-1-nitrosourea; NSC 409962

Molecular and structural information

Molecular formula: $C_5H_9Cl_2N_3O_2$

Molecular weight: 214

Structural formula:

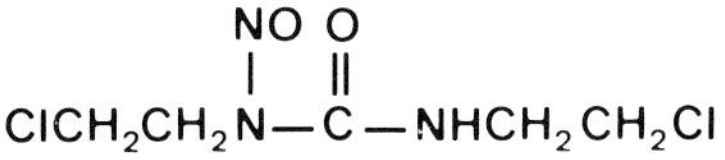

$$\underset{\displaystyle CICH_2CH_2N}{\overset{\displaystyle NO}{|}}\!-\!\underset{\displaystyle C}{\overset{\displaystyle O}{\|}}\!-\!NHCH_2CH_2Cl$$

Physical properties

Data obtained from Wade (1977) or Windholz (1983), unless otherwise specified

Description:	Light-yellow powder that melts to an oily liquid
Melting-point:	30–32 °C
Solubility:	Soluble in water (4 mg/ml) and 50% ethanol (150 mg/mL); soluble in ethanol (1 to 2); very soluble in lipids
Stability:	Both powders and liquids are stable; in aqueous solutions, most stable at pH 4 (half-life, 511 min); in acid solutions and in solutions above pH 7, decomposes rapidly (Loo *et al.*, 1966); at neutral pH, half-life is 98 min (Schein *et al.*, 1978)
Spectral data:	NMR spectra (Lown & Chauhan, 1981a) and MS spectra (Weinkam *et al.*, 1978) have been reported.

16. Semustine

Nomenclature

Chemical Abstracts Services Registry Number: 13909-09-6

Chemical Abstracts Name: Urea, N-(2-chloroethyl)-N'-(4-methylcyclohexyl)-N-nitroso-

Synonyms: ICIG 1110; Me-CCNU; methyl-CCNU; NSC 95441; urea, 1-(2-chlorethyl)-3-(4-methylcyclo-hexyl)-1-nitroso-

Molecular and structural information

Molecular formula: $C_{10}H_{18}ClN_3O_2$

Molecular weight: 247.7

Structural formula:

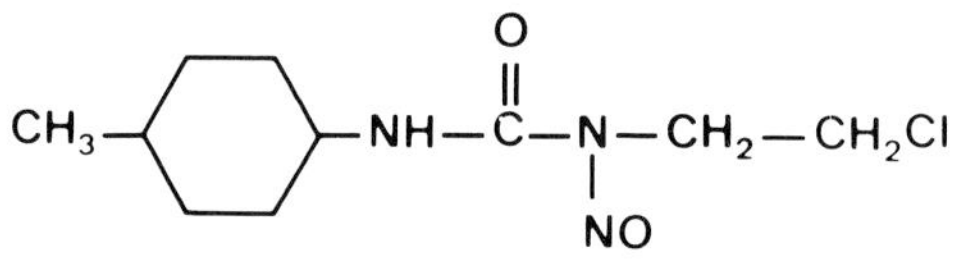

Physical properties

Data obtained from National Institutes of Health (private communication), unless otherwise mentioned

Description:	Light pale-yellow powder
Melting-point:	68–69 °C (Lown & Chauhan, 1981b)
Solubility:	0.09 mg/mL in water, 0.1 mol/L HCl or 0.1 mol/L NaOH; 0.1 mg/mL in 10% ethanol; 100 mg/mL in absolute ethanol; 250 mg/mL in dimethylsulfoxide
Stability:	Bulk sample stored at room temperature for 30 days showed 4% decomposition due to ultraviolet irradiation; solutions in 10% ethanol showed 2% decomposition after 6 h when refrigerated and 25% decomposition after 6 h at room temperature; solutions in methanol are unstable
Spectral data:	IR and NMR spectra have been presented (Lown & Chauhan, 1981b); UV λ_{max} 229 ± 2 nm.

17. PCNU

Nomenclature

Chemical Abstracts Services Registry Number: 13909-02-9

Chemical Abstracts Name: Urea, *N*-(2-chloroethyl)-*N'*-(2,6-dioxo-3-piperidinyl)-*N*-nitroso-

Synonyms: 1-(2-Chloroethyl)-3-(2,6-dioxo-3-piperidyl)-1-nitrosourea; NSC 95466; urea, 1-(2-chloroethyl)-3-(2,6-dioxo-3-piperidyl)-1-nitroso-

Molecular and structural information

Molecular formula: $C_8H_{11}ClN_4O_4$

Molecular weight: 262.7

Structural formula:

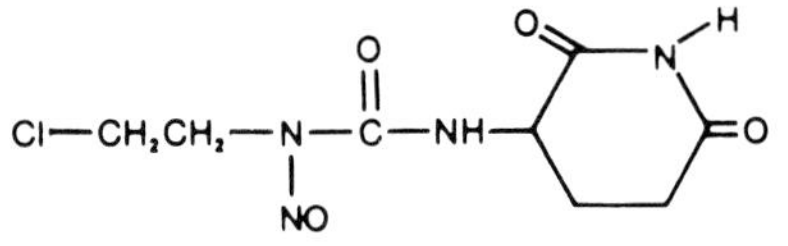

Physical properties

Data obtained from National Institutes of Health (private communication), unless otherwise mentioned

Description:	Fine, ivory powder
Solubility:	<1 mg/mL in water (National Cancer Institute, 1980); 2–3 mg/mL in buffer pH 9; 1 mg/mL in 10% ethanol; 2–3 mg/mL in 95% ethanol; 3–4 mg/mL in methanol; 1–3 mg/mL in chloroform; and 12.5–15 mg/mL in acetone
Stability:	Solution showed 38% decomposition after 24 h (National Cancer Institute, 1980); bulk sample stored at 60 °C for 10 days decomposed by 18%; bulk sample stable for 60 days at room temperature and daylight

18. Melphalan

Nomenclature

Chemical Abstracts Services Registry Number: 148-82-3

Chemical Abstracts Name: L-Phenylalanine, 4-[bis-(2-chloroethyl)amino]- (9th edition); alanine, 3-{p-[bis(-2-chloroethyl)amino]phenyl}- (8th edition)

Synonyms: Alkeran; CB 3025; 3025 C.B.; *p*-di(2-chloroethyl)amino-L-phenyl-alanine; levofalan; NSC-8806; PAM; L-PAM; phenylalanine mustard; L-phenyl-alanine mustard; phenylalanine nitrogen mustard; sarcoclorin; L-sarcolysin; L-sarcolysine; L-sarkolysin

Molecular and structural information

Molecular formula: $C_{13}H_{18}Cl_2N_2O_2$

Molecular weight: 305.2

Structural formula:

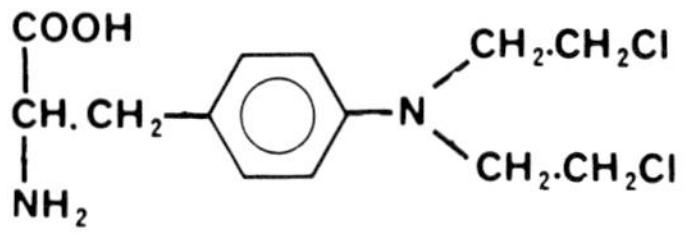

Physical properties

Data obtained from Wade (1977) or Windholz (1983), unless otherwise specified

Description: White, or almost white, odourless powder; needles from methanol

Melting-point: $\simeq 177\,^{\circ}C$ or $182{-}183\,^{\circ}C$ (decomposition); loses about 7% of its weight on drying

Optical rotation: $[\alpha]_D^{25} +7.5^{\circ}$ (C = 1.33 in 1.0 N HCl); $[\alpha]_D^{22} -31.5^{\circ}$ (C = 0.67 in methanol)

Solubility: Almost insoluble in water; soluble in ethanol, propylene glycol and dilute mineral acids; soluble at 1 in 150 in methanol; insoluble in chloroform and ether
                     For medical use, solutions are prepared by solubilizing 100 mg in 1 mL acid alcohol solvent and diluting to 10 mL with a phosphate buffer (final pH, $\simeq 7$) (National Cancer Institute, 1983)

Stability: Sensitive to air and light; should be stirred at temperatures not exceeding $25\,^{\circ}C$ in air-tight containers protected from light
                     Medical reconstitutions are poorly stable (National Cancer Institute, 1983)

Spectral data: Mass spectra have been reported (Pallante et al., 1980)
                     UV λ_{max} 260 nm, $E_1^1 = 560$ (in aqueous solutions at pH 7)

APPENDIX B
FURTHER REACTIONS OF ANTINEOPLASTIC AGENTS RELEVANT TO THEIR DEGRADATION

1. Biological methods

The biodegradation of antineoplastic agents has been studied very little, and only one reference was found in the literature (Table 2).

Table 2. Biological degradation of antineoplastic agents

Antineoplastic agent	Reaction products	Reaction and % conversion	Reference
Methotrexate	Pteroic acid	A pseudomonad that utilizes glutamate derived from the hydrolysis of methotrexate has been isolated. The enzyme responsible for the deamination has been partially purified; it has an optimal pH of 7.3 and a K_m towards methotrexate of $2.4 \ 10^{-4}$ M.	Levy & Goldman (1967)

2. Chemical methods

Table 3 presents data from studies on the stability and chemical reactions of antineoplastic agents that have been reported in the literature. The stability studies were carried out to test the reduction in activity of the compounds; loss of biological activity was not measured. However, some of the reactions might be of interest for establishing new degradation methods.

Table 3. Stability and chemical reactions of some antineoplastic agents

Antineoplastic agent	Reaction products	Reaction and % conversion	Reference
Daunorubicin	O-Trimethylsilyl derivative	Treatment by trimethylsilylimidazol/pyridine at 65°C for 10 min; quantitative yield	Andrews *et al.* (1982a)
Daunorubicin	A modified aglycone (in which ring A is deacetylated and aromatic) is the major degradation product after 10 min	UV irradiation of solutions in 50 mM NaCl, 50 mmol/L phosphate pH 7.05 produces precipitates which vary in quantity with the duration of irradiation and the presence or absence of oxygen	Gray & Phillips (1981)
Daunorubicin		Adsorption of 10^{-4} mol/L from saline solution by trisulfo-copper-phthalocyanine; 99% removal	Hayatsu *et al.* (1983)
Doxorubicin, methotrexate		Solutions of normal pharmacy standards are stable for up to 30 days when stored at $-20°C$ and when subjected to 5 thawings and refreezings	Karlsen *et al.* (1983)
Doxorubicin	Complexes with metals	Binding constants to Fe^{3+} and Cu^{2+} have been investigated	May *et al.* (1980)
Doxorubicin	Corresponding carboxylic acid	Cleavage at C_{13}–C_{14} bond by one equivalent of metaperiodate	Tong *et al.* (1976)
Doxorubicin		At concentrations below 500 µg/ml, appreciable photodegradation can occur	Tavoloni *et al.* (1980)
Doxorubicin		When reconstituted according to manufacturer's instructions, the resulting solution kept at room temperature and in daylight was stable both in glass and plastic containers	Benvenuto *et al.* (1981)
Carmustine		Chemical decomposition in 0.1 mol/L phosphate buffer pH (7.4) at 37°C occurs with a half-life of 40 min	Aukerman *et al.* (1983)
Carmustine		Half-life in 0.2 mol/L citric acid is about 270 h at 0°C and 16.9 at 20°C. Very slow decay in ethanol solution acidified with a drop of 1 mol/L citric acid per 10 mL. Half-life at 20°C is 250–300 h	Bartošek *et al.* (1978)
Carmustine		When reconstituted in ethanol/water at a concentration of 1.25 mg/mL, solutions undergo 10% degradation in glass containers at pH 4.6 in 7.7 h and in plastic containers at pH 4.2 in 0.6 h	Benvenuto *et al.* (1981)

Antineoplastic agent	Reaction products	Reaction and % conversion	Reference
Carmustine	At pH 5.0: ethylene glycol and acetaldehyde; at pH 7.4: chloroethanol and acetaldehyde	Incubation of 0.05 mol/L solutions at 37 °C in 0.1 mol/L sodium phosphate buffer pH 5.0 or 7.4 leads to decomposition	Brundrett (1980)
Semustine	2-(2-Chloro-ethyl)-4-(trans-4-methylcyclo-hexyl)semicar-bazide	Treatment of an ethereal solution with sodium tetrahydroborate (III) in presence of ethanol for 20 min at room temperature leads to decomposition	Caddy & Idowu (1982b)
Semustine	1-(2-Chloro-ethyl)-3-(trans-4-methylcyclo-hexyl)urea	Denitrosation by peroxiacetic acid	Caddy & Idowu (1982a)
Carmustine	Acetaldeyhde (31%); dichloro-ethane (2%); chloroethanol (63%); vinyl chloride (4%)	Decomposition of solutions in 0.05 mol/L sodium cacodylate buffer (pH 7) containing 0.1 mol/L sodium chloride	Colvin et al. (1974)
Carmustine	Vinyl chloride (2%); acetal-dehyde (26%); dichloroethane (2%); chloro-ethanol (71%)	Decomposition of solution in 0.1 mol/L phosphate buffer (pH 7.4) at 37 °C	Colvin et al. (1976)
Lomustine	Vinyl chloride (4%); acetal-dehyde (37%); dichloroethane (3%); chloro-ethanol (56%)		
Carmustine		When in solution in 5% dextrose and 0.9% sodium chloride, no decomposition occurs within 90 min; addition of sodium carbonate increases the rate of degradation (only 73% remaining after 90 min)	Colvin et al. (1980)
Streptozotocin	Diazomethane	Treatment with 2 mol/L sodium hydroxide at 0 °C leads to decomposition with evolution of diazomethane	Herr et al. (1967)
Streptozotocin		5 µg/ml solution in cell culture medium incubated at 37 °C in an atmosphere of 8% CO_2 in air; half-life, 19 min	Jensen et al. (1977)

Antineoplastic agent	Reaction products	Reaction and % conversion	Reference
Carmustine		Stability evaluated in various buffers (citrate, acetate, phosphate, barbital) over a pH range of 3–8; minimum degradation rate obtained between pH 5.2 and 5.5; rate increases rapidly with pH between pH 5.5 and 8	Laskar & Ayres (1977a)
Carmustine		Rate of degradation investigated in ethanol, propylene glycol, dimethylsulfoxide, mannitol and aqueous solutions of these solvents. The aqueous solvent mixtures containing the least water demonstrated minimal degradation rates	Laskar & Ayres (1977b)
Carmustine		Stability evaluated in a range of buffer pH 1–9.3; most stable at pH 4; decomposes rapidly in acid and even more rapidly in alkali; $T^{1/2}$ are given over the range of pH	Loo *et al.* (1966)
Carmustine	1-Bromo-2-chloroethane; 2-bromoethanol	Decomposition in a saturated sodium bromide solution pH 7.2, at 37°C in a sealed tube for 24 h	Lown *et al.* (1979)
Carmustine	Ethanol from acetaldehyde intermediate	Decomposition in phosphate buffer at pH 7.1 and 25°C in 99% $H_2{}^{18}O$ in presence of alcohol dehydrogenase and NADH	Lown & Chauhan (1982)
Carmustine; lomustine		Carmustine had a half-life of 9 days in sesame oil, 30 days in propylene glycol and 74 days in 95% ethanol	Montgomery *et al.* (1967)
	N_2-2-Chloroethanol; 2-chloroethylisocyanate 1,3-Bis(2-chloroethyl)urea; 2-chloroethanol	When refluxed in 2,2,4-trimethylpentane, for 1 h under anhydrous conditions, carmustine decomposes completely Decomposition of carmustine by heating an aqueous solution at 50°C for 96 h	
	1,3-Bis(2-chloroethyl)urea	Decomposition of carmustine in water containing the same molar amount of triethylamine, by stirring for 1 h at 5–10°C and 18 h at room temperature	
	1-(2-Chloroethyl)-3-cyclohexyl urea 2-(2-Chloroethylamino)-2-oxazoline hydrochloride	Decomposition of carmustine in water containing the same molar amount of cyclohexylamine, by stirring for 1 h at 5°C and 2 h at 10°C Decomposition of carmustine in phosphate buffer, pH 7.2	
		Half-lives of carmustine and lomustine in water and in various buffers are presented.	

Antineoplastic agent	Reaction products	Reaction and % conversion	Reference
Carmustine, lomustine, chlorozotocin	Acetaldehyde; 2-chloroethanol; chloride ion	Stability of all three nitrosoureas has been tested in boiled distilled water, phosphate buffer pH 7, acetate buffer pH 7, tris buffer pH 7.4, dioxane:boiled distilled water (1:2), dioxane:phosphate buffer pH 7 (1:2) and phosphate buffer pH 7.4. Decomposition is dependent on buffering at or near physiological pH. Ratio of products is presented	Montgomery et al. (1975)
Carmustine, lomustine		Stability of solutions in 0.5 mol/L cacodylate buffer (pH 7.0) containing 3.3% dimethylsulfoxide has been studied at 37°C: T½ carmustine, 81.3 min; T½ lomustine, 103 min	Morimoto et al. (1978)
Carmustine, lomustine, semustine	2-Chloroethanol (a); chloride ion (b); acetaldehyde (c)	Degradation study in phosphate buffer (pH 7.4) at 37°C in 3 h: Carmustine: a, 50%, b, 50%, c, 11%; Lomustine: a, 35%, b, 65%, c, 19%; Semustine: a, 34%, b, 65%, c, 24%	Nakamura et al. (1979)
Carmustine, lomustine		Stability study in phosphate buffered saline pH 7.4 (145 mmol/L sodium chloride, 10 mmol/L sodium phosphate) at 37°C: T½ carmustine, 98 min; T½ lomustine, 117 min	Panasci et al. (1977)
Lomustine, semustine	2-Chloroethanol; acetaldehyde; vinyl chloride; ethylene; cyclohexylamine	Stability study in 0.1 mol/L phosphate buffer pH 7.4 at 37°C: T½ lomustine, 48 min; T½ semustine, 70 min	Reed et al. (1975)
Carmustine, lomustine, chlorozotocin		Stability study in phosphate buffered saline pH 7.4: T½ carmustine, 98 min; T½ lomustine, 117 min; T½ chlorozotocin, 48 min	Schein et al. (1978)
Lomustine		Rate of hydrolysis higher with increasing hydroxide ion concentration within pH ranges 7–8; decomposition rate reduced at lower pHs but reduction in rate is lower	Yoshida & Yano (1982)
Chlorozotocin	Acetaldehyde; 2-chloroethanol; other products	Decomposition in aqueous solution at various pHs and buffer concentrations at 37°C follows first-order kinetics from pH 2 and above; the higher the pH the greater the rate of decomposition.	Chatterji et al. (1978)
Cyclophosphamide	Acrolein; others	Oxidation of 28 μmol/L by H_2O_2, $FeSO_4$, $FeSO_4$-EDTA, $FeSO_4$-EDTA-H_2O_2, $FeSO_4$-EDTA-ascorbic acid, $FeSO_4$-EDTA-ascorbic acid-H_2O_2 or $CuSO_4$-sodium ascorbate produces 0.07 to 5.0 μmol acrolein	Alarcon & Meienhoffer (1971)
Cyclophosphamide		When reconstituted with sterile water, a solution kept at room temperature and in daylight was stable in glass and plastic containers for at least 24 h	Benvenuto et al. (1981)

Antineoplastic agent	Reaction products	Reaction and % conversion	Reference
Cyclophosphamide		When heated for 15 min at 50 °C or 60 °C, the potency of aqueous solutions did not change appreciably; at 70 °C, only 90.2% recovered and at 80 °C only 77.5%	Brooke *et al.* (1975)
Cyclophosphamide		Solutions in parenteral liquids at 24–27 °C or 5 °C are unstable on prolonged storage; solutions are more stable at 5 °C than at room temperature. First-order rates of reaction have been found, and the rate constants are presented under various conditions	Brooke *et al.* (1973a)
Cyclophosphamide		Solutions in aromatic elixir USP are unstable on prolonged storage at 45 °C, 35 °C or room temperature. First-order reaction rate has been demonstrated in all cases; greatly reduced at 5 °C, as expected from Arrhenius equation	Brooke *et al.* (1973b)
Cyclophosphamide		Complete destruction is obtained in 0.2 mol/L potassium hydroxide in methanol in less than 1 h	Ehrenberg & Wachtmeister (1977)
Cyclophosphamide	N-(2-Hydroxy-ethyl)-N'-(3-hydroxypropyl)-ethylenediamine; N-(3-hydroxy-propyl)-piperazine	Boiling for several hours leads to hydrolysis; initially, an intramolecular alkylation occurs, followed by a sequence of simple hydrolytic cleavage of P-N and P-O bonds	Friedman (1967); Friedman *et al.* (1965)
Cyclophosphamide		0.4% solutions in sodium chloride injection are stable for at least 4 weeks at refrigerator temperature	Gallelli (1967)
Cyclophosphamide	4-Ketocyclo-phosphamide; monodechloro-ethylated derivative	Treatment of 5 mg of compound with 10 mg $KMnO_4$ in 0.2 mL water at 20 °C for 4 h (98.5% removal) or in 0.2 mL acetone at 20 °C for 3 h (22% removal)	Jarman (1973)
Ifosfamide	2-(1-Aziridinyl)-3-(2-chloro-ethyl)-2H-1,3,2-oxazaphosphori-nane-2-oxide	Reaction of 1.2 mmol sodium hydride in ether with 1 mmol ifosfamide in benzene for 24 h results in 100% removal	Ludeman *et al.* (1979)
Cyclophosphamide	N',N-Bis(2-chlo-roethyl)diamido-phosphoric acid (2-carboxyethyl-ester)	Treatment of 280 mg in 30 mL water with 210 mg $KMnO_4$ at 4 °C after pH adjustment to 2.5 with 0.1 mol/L HCl results in decomposition	Norpoth *et al.* (1972)
Cyclophosphamide	4-Hydroxycyclo-phosphamide	Oxidation with Fenton reagent (1:1 or 1:1.5 $FeSO_4$:H_2O_2)	Van der Steen *et al.* (1973)

Antineoplastic agent	Reaction products	Reaction and % conversion	Reference
Cyclophosphamide	4-Peroxycyclo-phosphamide 4-hydroperoxycy-clophosphamide	Treatment of 1 g in 30 mL water containing 1.25 g $FeSO_4.7H_2O$ at 5 °C with 0.5 mL 30% H_2O_2 yields two products, which react chemically as both aldehydes and alkylating agents	Struck et al. (1974)
Cyclophosphamide	4-Ketocyclophos-phamide; 4-hy-droxycyclo-phosphamide anhydro-dimer	Oxidation with Fenton reagent in phosphate buffer solution (pH 6.4) for 2 h at 0–10 °C	Takamizawa et al. (1974)
Cyclophosphamide	Acrolein	Oxidation of 28 µmol with a Fenton oxidation system ($FeSO_4$ 30 µmol, EDTA 53 µmol in 5 mL 0.1 mol/L phosphate buffer and 100 µl 5% H_2O_2) for 3 h at 37 °C	Thomson & Colvin (1974)
Cyclophosphamide		When heated at 60, 75 or 90 °C, decomposes following a first-order rate of reaction; hydrolysis is independent of pH except at pH <1 or >11	Masaharu et al. (1967)
Methotrexate		Irradiation by 4000, 8000 and 12 000 Lux lamps of aqueous solutions containing 2.5, 1 or 0.5 mg/mL provokes photodegradation; the more diluted the solution, the more efficient the degradation	Battelli et al. (1983)
Methotrexate		Solutions kept at room temperature and daylight in glass or plastic containers are stable for at least 24 h	Benvenuto et al. (1981)
Methotrexate	N^{10}-Methyl-pteroylglutamic acid 2,4-Diamino-6-pteridinecarbal-dehyde; 2,4-diamino-6-pteridine carboxylic acid; p-aminoben-zoylglutamic acid	At pHs above 7, methotrexate is hydrolysed at 85 °C, following first-order kinetics; rate increases with pH. Half-life varies from 13 days at pH 8.5 to 0.038 days at pH 12 Methotrexate in solution undergoes slow photolytic degradation catalysed by the presence of bicarbonate ions	Chatterji & Gallelli (1978)
Methotrexate	N^{10}-Methyl-pteroylglutamic acid	At pHs above 6.5, methotrexate is hydrolysed at 85 °C, following first-order kinetics; rate increases with pH. At pHs below 6.5, route of degradation was much more complex	Hansen et al. (1983)
Methotrexate		Solutions in 5% dextrose with 0.05 mEq/mL of sodium bicarbonate decompose by 1.4% in 72 h and 6.1% in 7 days when stored at 4–5 °C and protected from light; and by 6.2% in 72 h and 14.9% in 7 days when stored at room temperature, not protected from light	Humphreys et al. (1978)

Antineoplastic agent	Reaction products	Reaction and % conversion	Reference
Methotrexate		Solutions of normal pharmacy standards are stable up to 30 days when stored at $-20\,°C$ and when subjected to 5 thawings and refreezings	Karlsen *et al.* (1983)
Dichlorometho-trexate		Solutions in bacteriostatic 0.9% NaCl containing 200 U/mL heparin showed no appreciable decomposition in control vials for up to 28 days	Keller & Ensminger (1982)
Cisplatin		Stable in solutions in physiological saline for at least 24 h; in presence of dextrose, two unidentified breakdown products are formed in less than 2 h in the dark, at room temperature	Earhart (1978, 1979)
Cisplatin		Solutions in 0.9% saline degrade 3% in <1 h and are then stable for at least 24 h at room temperature; exposure to strong fluorescent light creates major differences in the entire UV absorption spectrum, but little change is noticeable when exposed to normal room light.	Greene *et al.* (1979)
Cisplatin		In aqueous solutions, the presence of sodium chloride enhances the stability of cisplatin; dextrose or mannitol does not affect the stability of the drug; sodium bicarbonate adversely affects the stability significantly. Normal laboratory light has no effect on stability.	Hincal *et al.* (1979); Repta *et al.* (1979)
Cisplatin		Stable for 8 h at $25\,°C$ in 5% dextrose with 0.45% NaCl and 1.875% mannitol or 5% dextrose with 0.33% NaCl and 1.875% mannitol; stable for 72 h in 5% dextrose in 0.33% NaCl containing 20 mg KCl with 1.875% mannitol, in bacteriostatic water for injection with benzyl alcohol USP, in bacteriostatic water for injection with parabens USP, or in mixtures of the above solutions	Mariani *et al.* (1980)
Vincristine sulfate		When reconstituted with bacteriostatic sodium chloride, solutions kept at room temperature and in daylight are stable in glass containers for at least 24 h but degraded by 10% in plastic containers within 10 h.	Benvenuto *et al.* (1981)
Vinblastine sulfate		When reconstituted with sodium chloride injection USP, a solution kept at room temperature and in daylight is stable both in glass and plastic containers for at least 24 h.	
Vinblastine sulfate	Vincristine	Oxidation of vinblastine sulfate with chromic acid or its salt at low temperature produces vincristine in 50% yield.	Jovanovics *et al.* (1975)
Vinblastine sulfate		Solutions in bacteriostatic 0.9% sodium chloride are degraded by 20% in control vials in 14 days	Keller & Ensminger (1982)

Antineoplastic agent	Reaction products	Reaction and % conversion	Reference
6-Mercaptopurine	Purine-6-sulfuric acid	Treatment of a deoxygenated methanolic solution with a solution of *m*-chloroperoxy benzoic acid in methanol in a nitrogen atmosphere results in 20–25% conversion.	Abraham *et al.* (1983)
6-Mercaptopurine	Potassium purine-6-sulfonate	Treatment of an aqueous/ethanol (50%) solution with 0.05 mol/L potassium permanganate results in 57% formation of the sulfonate.	Brown & Hoskins (1972)
6-Mercaptopurine, 6-thioguanine		Suspensions of 6-mercaptopurine (50 mg/mL) or 6-thioguanine (40 mg/mL) in a mixture of cologel and flavouring agent stored at room temperature kept over 90% of their potency for 14 days (6-mercaptopurine) or 84 days (6-thioguanine)	Dressman & Poust (1983)
Melphalan		Suspensions in a mixture of cologel and flavouring agent are very unstable: >80% degradation after 1 day and 100% after 4 days of storage at room temperature, and >50% degradation after 7 days' storage at 5°C	Dressman & Poust (1983)
Melphalan		Stability tested at 37°C in 0.9% NaCl, 0.156 mol/L HCl pH 1.7, 0.013 mol/L HCl, 0.013 mol/L H_3PO_4 and 0.06 mol/L phosphate buffers; chloride ion favours stability, while phosphate favours decomposition (95% degradation in 3 h in 0.06 mol/L phosphate buffer	Chang *et al.* (1979)
Melphalan	4-[2(-Chloro-ethyl) (2-hy-droxyethyl)-amino]-L-phenyl-alanine; 4-[bis(2-hydroxyethyl)-amino]-L-phenyl-alanine	Rate of hydrolysis studied in various buffers (pH 3–9) in presence or absence of chloride ion: most stable at low pH; chloride ions reduce the rate of hydrolysis	Flora *et al.* (1979)
Melphalan		Stability of melphalan bound to albumin is about 3 times higher than unbound in solution	Ehrsson & Lönroth (1982)

REFERENCES

Abraham, R.T., Benson, L.M. & Jardine, I. (1983) Synthesis and pH dependent stability of purine-6-sulfenic acid, a putative reactive metabolite of 6-thiopurine. *J. med. Chem., 26,* 1523–1526

Akedo, H. & Shinkai, K. (1982) Isotachophoretic determination of adriamycin and adriamycinol in human plasma. *J. Chromatogr., 227,* 262–265

Akira, Y., Yoshimi, M., Hiroe, K., Noboru, O., Eiichi, H., Hideki, H. & Tetsuya, M. (1982) Enzyme immunoassay of methotrexate in blood and its stability in infusion solutions. *Byoin. Yakugaku, 8(5),* 354–358

Akpofure, C., Riley, C.A., Sinkole, J.A. & Evans, W.E. (1982) Quantitation of daunorubicin and its metabolites by high performance liquid chromatography with electrochemical detection. *J. Chromatogr., 232,* 377–383

Alarcon, R.A. & Meienhoffer, J. (1971) Formation of the cytotoxic aldehyde acrolein during *in vitro* degradation of cyclophosphamide. *Nature-New Biol., 233,* 250–252

American Society of Hospital Pharmacists (1985) Technical assistance bulletin on handling cytotoxic drugs in hospital. *Am. J. Hosp. Pharm., 42,* 131–137

Ames, B.N., McCann, J. & Yamaski, E. (1975) Methods for detecting carcinogens and mutagens with the *Salmonella*/mammalian-microsome mutagenicity test. *Mutat. Res., 31,* 347–364

Anderson, R., Dona, W. & Ruckett, W. (1982) Risk of handling injectable antineoplastic agents. *Am. J. Hosp. Pharm., 39,* 1881–1887

Andrews, P.A., Brenner, D.E., Chou, F.-T.E., Kubo, H. & Bachur, N.R. (1980) Facile and definitive determination of human adriamycin and daunorubicin metabolites by high pressure liquid chromatography. *Drug Metab. Disposition, 8(3),* 152–156

Andrews, P.A., Callery, P.S., Chou, F.-T.E., May, M.E. & Bachur, N.R. (1982a) Qualitative analysis of trimethylsilylated daunosamine and N-alkylated analogs by gas chromatography/mass spectrometry. *Anal. Biochem., 126,* 258–267

Andrews, P.A., Egorin, M.J., May, M.E. & Bachur, N.R. (1982b) Reversed phase high performance liquid chromatography analysis of 6-thioguanine applicable to pharmacologic studies in humans. *J. Chromatogr., 227,* 83–91

Arcamone, F., Cassinelli, G., Fantini, G., Grein, A., Orezzi, P., Pol, C. & Spalla, C. (1969) Adriamycin, 14-hydroxidaunomycin, a new antitumour antibiotic from *S. peucetius* var. caesius. *Biotech. Bioeng., 11,* 1101–1110

Arcamone, F., Penco, S. & Vigevani, A. (1975) Adriamycin (NSC-123127): New chemical developments and analogs. *Cancer Chemother. Rep., 6(2),* 123–129

Aukerman, S.L., Brundrett, R.B., Hilton, J. & Hartman, P.E. (1983) Effect of plasma and carboxylesterase on the stability, mutagenicity, and DNA cross-linking activity of some direct-acting *N*-nitroso compounds. *Cancer Res., 43,* 175–181

Baker, C.E., Jr (1980) *Physicians' Desk Reference*, 34th ed., Oradell, NJ, Medical Economics Co., pp. 708–709

Bannister, S.J., Sternson, L.A. & Repta, A.J. (1979) Urine analysis of platinum species derived from cis-dichlorodiammineplatinum (II) by high-performance liquid chromatography following derivatization with diethyldithiocarbamate. *J. Chromatogr., 173,* 333–342

Bannister, S.J., Sternson, L.A. & Repta, A.J. (1983) Evaluation of reductive amperometric detection in the liquid chromatographic determination of antineoplastic platinum complexes. *J. Chromatogr., 273,* 301–318

Bartsch, H., Malaveille, C., Camus, A.M., Martel-Planche, G., Brun, G., Hautefeuille, A., Sabadie, N., Barbin, A., Kuroki, T., Drevon, C., Piccoli, C. & Montesano, R. (1980) Validation and comparative studies on 180 chemicals with *S. typhimurium* strains and V79 Chinese hamster cells in the presence of various metabolising systems. *Mutat. Res., 31,* 347–364

Bartosěk, I. & Cattaneo, M.T. (1982) *Electrochemical determination of submicrogram quantities of cis-diamminedichloroplatinum (II) in biological samples.* In: Periti, P. & Gialdroni, G.G., eds, *Current Chemotherapy Immunotherapy,* pp. 1382–1383

Bartosěk, I., Daniel, S. & Sýkora, S. (1978) Differential pulse polarographic determination of submicrogram quantities of carmustine and related compounds in biological samples. *J. pharm. Sci., 67(8),* 1160–1163

Bartosěk, I., Cattaneo, M.T., Grasselli, G., Guaitani, A., Urso, R., Zucca, E., Libretti, A. & Garattini, S. (1983) Polarographic assay of submicrogram quantities of cis-dichlorodiammineplatinum (II) in biological samples. *Tumori, 69,* 395–402

Battelli, G., Marra, M., Romagnoli, E., Tagliapietra, L. & Tassara, A. (1983) Fotosensibilità di soluzioni acquose di methotrexate e di acido ascorbico. *Boll. Chim. Farm., 123,* 149–157

Benezra, S.A. & Foss, P.R.B. (1978) *6-Mercaptopurine.* In: Florey, K., ed., *Analytical Profiles of Drug Substances*, Vol. 7, New York, Academic Press, pp. 343–357

Benvenuto, J.A., Anderson, R.W., Kerkof, K., Smith, R.G. & Loo Ti Li (1981) Stability and compatibility of anti-tumour agents in glass and plastic containers. *Am. J. Hosp. Pharm., 38,* 1914–1918

Bolanowska, W., Gessner, T. & Priesler, H. (1983) A simplified method for determination of daunorubicin, adriamycin and their chief fluorescent metabolites in human plasma by high pressure liquid chromatography. *Cancer Chemother. Pharmacol., 10,* 187–191

Bosanquet, A.G. & Gilby, E.D. (1982) Measurement of plasma melphalan at therapeutic concentrations using isocratic high performance liquid chromatography. *J. Chromatogr., 232,* 345–354

Bots, A.M.B., Van Oort, W.J. & Noordhoek, J. (1983) Analysis of adriamycin and adriamycinol in micro volumes of rat plasma. *J. Chromatogr., 272,* 421–427

Boughton, O.D., Brown, R.D., Bryant, R., Burger, F.J. & Combs, C.M. (1972) Assay of cyclophosphamide. *J. Pharm. Sci., 61(1)*, 97–100

Bower, E.L.Y. & Winefordner, J.D. (1978) Room temperature phosphorescence characteristics and limits of detection of several pharmaceutical compounds. *Anal. chim. Acta, 101*, 319–332

Brabec, V., Vrána, O. & Kleinwächter, V. (1983) Determination of platinum in biological material by differential pulse polarography: Analysis in urine, plasma and tissue following sample combustion. *Coll. Czech. Commun., 48(10)*, 2903–2908

Breithaupt, H. & Goebel, G. (1981) Quantitative high performance liquid chromatography of 6-thioguanine in biological fluids. *J. chromatogr. Sci., 19*, 496–499

Breithaupt, H., Küenzlen, E. & Goebel, G. (1982) Rapid high-pressure liquid chromatographic determination of methotrexate and its metabolites 7-hydroxymethotrexate and 2,4-diamino-N^{10}-methylpteroic acid in biological fluids. *Anal. Biochem., 121*, 103–113

Brooke, D., Bequette, R.J. & Davis, R.E. (1973a) Chemical stability of cyclophosphamide in parenteral solutions. *Am. J. Hosp. Pharm., 30*, 134–137

Brooke, D., Davis, R.E. & Bequette, R.J. (1973b) Chemical stability of cyclophosphamide in aromatic elixir USP. *Am. J. Hosp. Pharm., 30*, 618–620

Brooke, D., Scott, J.A. & Bequette, R.J. (1975) Effect of briefly heating cyclophosphamide solutions. *Am. J. Hosp. Pharm., 32*, 44–45

Brown, D.J. & Hoskins, J.A. (1972) The preparation and reactivity of some potassium purine-, quinazoline-, and tetrahydroquinazoline-sulphonates. *Aust. J. Chem., 25*, 2641–2649

Brown, J.E., Wilkinson, P.A. & Brown, J.R. (1981) Rapid high-performance liquid chromatographic assay for the anthracyclines daunorubicin and 7-con-O-methylnogarol in plasma. *J. Chromatogr., 226*, 521–525

Brundrett, R.B. (1980) Chemistry of nitrosoureas. Intermediacy of 4,5-dihydro-1,2,3-oxadiazole in 1,3-bis(2-chloroethyl)-1-nitrosourea decomposition. *J. med. Chem., 23*, 1245–1247

Burns, J.H. (1972) *Vincristine sulfate and vinblastine sulfate*. In: Florey, K., ed., *Analytical Profiles of Drug Substances*, Vol. 1, New York, Academic Press, pp. 443–462, 463–480

Caddy, B. & Idowu, O.R. (1982a) Gas chromatographic determination of 1-(2-chloroethyl)-3-(*trans*-4-methylcyclohexyl)-1-nitrosourea(methyl-CCN). Part III. Denitrosation to the parent urea. *Analyst, 107*, 556–565

Caddy, B. & Idowu, O.R. (1982b) Gas chromatographic determination of 1-(2-chloroethyl)-3-(*trans*-4-methylcyclohexyl)-1-nitrosourea(methyl-CCN). Part II. Reduction to semicarbazide with sodium tetrahydroborate (III). *Analyst, 107*, 550–555

Cairnes, D.A. & Evans, W.E. (1982) High-performance liquid chromatographic assay of methotrexate, 7-hydroxymethotrexate, 4-deoxy-4-amino-N^{10}-methyl-pteroic acid and sulfamethoxazole in serum and cerebrospinal fluid. *J. Chromatogr., 231,* 103–110

Cano, J., Catalin, J. & Bues-Charbit, M. (1982) Platinum determination in plasma and urine by flameless atomic absorption spectrophotometry. *J. appl. Toxicol., 2(1),* 33–38

Castegnaro, M., Hunt, D.C., Sansone, E.B., Schuller, P.L., Siriwardana, M.G., Telling, G.M., Van Egmond, H.P. & Walker, E.A. (1980) *Laboratory Decontamination and Destruction of Aflatoxins, B$_1$, B$_2$, G$_1$, G$_2$ in Laboratory Wastes (IARC Scientific Publications No. 37),* Lyon, International Agency for Research on Cancer

Castegnaro, M., Eisenbrand, G., Ellen, G., Keefer, L., Klein, D., Sansone, E.B., Spincer, D., Telling, G.M. & Webb, K. (1982) *Laboratory Decontamination and Destruction of Carcinogens in Laboratory Wastes: Some N-Nitrosamines (IARC Scientific Publications No. 43),* Lyon, International Agency for Research on Cancer

Castegnaro, M., Grimmer, G., Hutzinger, O., Karcher, W., Kunte, H., Lafontaine, M., Sansone, E.B., Telling, G.M. & Tucker, S.P. (1983a) *Laboratory Decontamination and Destruction of Carcinogens in Laboratory Wastes: Some Polycyclic Aromatic Hydrocarbons (IARC Scientific Publications No. 49),* Lyon, International Agency for Research on Cancer

Castegnaro, M., Ellen, G., Lafontaine, M., van der Plas, H.C., Sansone, E.B. & Tucker, S.P. (1983b) *Laboratory Decontamination and Destruction of Carcinogens in Laboratory Wastes: Some Hydrazines (IARC Scientific Publications No. 54),* Lyon, International Agency for Research on Cancer

Castegnaro, M., Benard, M., van Broekhoven, L.W., Fine, D., Massey, R., Sansone, E.B., Smith, P.L.R., Spiegelhalder, B., Stacchini, A., Telling, G.M. & Vallon, J.J. (1983c) *Laboratory Decontamination and Destruction of Carcinogens in Laboratory Wastes: Some N-Nitrosamides (IARC Scientific Publications No. 55),* Lyon, International Agency for Research on Cancer

Castegnaro, M., Barek, J., Dennis, J., Ellen, G., Klibanov, M., Lafontaine, M., Mitchum, R., Van Roosmalen, P., Sansone, E.B., Sternson, L.A. & Vahl, M. (1985) *Laboratory Decontamination and Destruction of Carcinogens in Laboratory Wastes: Some Aromatic Amines and 4-Nitrobiphenyl (IARC Scientific Publications No. 64),* Lyon, International Agency for Research on Cancer

Chamberlin, A.R., Cheung, A.P.K. & Lim, P. (1976) *Methotrexate.* In: Florey, K., ed., *Analytical Profiles of Drug Substances,* Vol. 5, New York, Academic Press, pp. 283–306

Chang, Y., Sternson, L.A. & Repta, A.J. (1978) Development of a specific analytical method for cis-dichlorodiamineplatinum (II) in plasma. *Anal. Lett., B11(6),* 449–459

Chang, S.Y., Evans, T.L. & Alberts, D.S. (1979) The stability of melphalan in the presence of chloride ion. *Pharm. Pharmacol., 31,* 853–854

Chatterji, D.C. & Gallelli, J.F. (1977) High-pressure liquid chromatographic analysis of methotrexate in presence of its degradation products. *J. pharm. Sci., 66(9),* 1219–1222

Chatterji, D.C. & Gallelli, J.F. (1978) Thermal and photolytic decomposition of methotrexate in aqueous solutions. *J. pharm. Sci., 67(4),* 526–531

Chatterji, D.C., Greene, R.F. & Gallelli, J.F. (1978) Mechanism of hydrolysis of halogenated nitrosourea. *J. pharm. Sci., 67(11),* 1527–1532

Chen, M.-L. & Chiou, W.L. (1981) Sensitive and rapid high performance liquid chromatographic method for the simultaneous determination of methotrexate and its metabolites in plasma, saliva and urine. *J. Chromatogr., 226,* 125–134

Colvin, M., Cowens, J.W., Brundrett, R.B., Kramer, B.S. & Ludlum, D.B. (1974) Decomposition of BCNU (1,3-bis(2-chloroethyl)-1-nitrosourea) in aqueous solution. *Biochem. biophys. Res. Commun., 60(2),* 515–520

Colvin, M., Brundrett, R.B., Cowens, J.W., Jardine, I. & Ludlum, D.B. (1976) A chemical basis for the antitumor activity of chloroethyl nitrosoureas. *Biochem. Pharmacol., 25,* 695–699

Colvin, M., Hartner, J. & Summerfield, M. (1980) Stability of carmustine in the presence of sodium carbonate. *Am. J. Hosp. Pharm., 37,* 677–678

Cone, N.J., Miller, R. & Neuss, N. (1963) Alkaloids of *Vinca rosea* Linn. (*Catharanthus roseus* G. Don). XV. Analysis of vinca alkaloids by thin layer chromatography. *J. pharm. Sci., 52(7),* 688–692

Daldrup, T., Susanto, F. & Michalke, P. (1981) Kombination von DC, GC (OV1 und OV17) und HPLC (RP18) zur schnellen Erkennung von Arzneimitteln, Rauschmitteln und verwandten Verbindungen. *Fresenius' Z. anal. Chem., 308,* 413–427

Davis, M.R. (1981) The Society of Hospital Pharmacists of Australia: Guidelines for safe handling of cytotoxic drugs in pharmacy departments and hospital wards. *Hosp. Pharm., 16,* 17–20

De Abreu, A., Van Baal, J.M., Schouten, T.J. & Schretlen, E. (1982) High performance liquid chromatographic determination of plasma 6-mercaptopurine in clinically relevant concentrations. *J. Chromatogr., 227,* 526–533

De Bruin, E.A., Tjaden, U.R., Van Oosterom, A.T., Leeflang, P. & Leclercq, P.A. (1983) Determination of the underivatized antineoplastic drugs cyclophosphamide and 5-fluorouracil and some of their metabolites by capillary gas chromatography combined with electron-capture and nitrogen-phosphorus selective detection. *J. Chromatogr., 279,* 603–608

Dressman, J.B. & Poust, R.L. (1983) Stability of allopurinol and five antineoplastics in suspension. *Am. J. Hosp. Pharm., 40,* 616–618

Dryhurst, G. (1969) Analytical utilization of polarographic and voltammetric behaviour of some sulphur containing purines. *Anal. chim. Acta, 47,* 275–284

Dusonchet, L., Gebbia, N. & Gerbasi, F. (1971) Spectrofluorimetric characterization of adriamycin, a new anti-tumour drug. *Pharmacol. Res. Commun., 3,* 55–65

Dutrieu, J. & Delmotte, Y.A. (1983) HPLC determination of methotrexate in serum or plasma optimized with a dual coulometric detector. *Fresenius' Z. Anal. Chem., 315,* 539–542

Earhart, R.H. (1978) Instability of cis-dichlorodiamineplatinum in dextrose solution. *Cancer Treatment Rep., 62(7),* 1105–1106

Earhart, R.H. (1979) Cis-dichlorodiamineplatinum (II) stability in aqueous vehicles. 'Authors response'. *Cancer Treatment Rep., 63(2),* 230–231

Egan, W., Jones, C.R. & McCluskey, M. (1981) Method for the measurement of melphalan in biological samples by high performance liquid chromatography with fluorescence detection. *J. Chromatogr., 224,* 338–342

Ehrenberg, L. & Wachtmeister, C.A. (1977) *Safety precautions in work with mutagenic and carcinogenic chemicals.* In: Kilbey, B.J., Legator, M., Nicols, W. & Ramel, C., eds, *Handbook of Mutagenicity Test Procedures,* Amsterdam, Elsevier, pp. 401–410

Ehrsson, H. & Lönroth, V. (1982) Degradation of melphalan in aqueous solutions. Influence of human albumin binding. *J. pharm. Sci., 71(7),* 826–827

Eisenbrand, G. & Habs, M. (1980) Chronic toxicity and carcinogenicity of cytostatic *N*-nitroso-(2-chloroethyl) ureas after repeated intravenous application to rats. *Dev. Toxicol. environ. Sci., 8,* 273–278

Eisenbrand, G., Habs, M., Zeller, W.J., Fiebig, H., Berger, M., Zelesny, O. & Schmael, D. (1981) New nitrosoureas – therapeutic and long term toxic effects of selected compounds in comparison to established drugs. *INSERM Symp., Vol. 19, ISS Nitrosourea Cancer Treat.,* 175–191

Eksborg, S. (1978) *Extraction properties and liquid chromatographic separation of adriamycin and daunorubicin and their hydroxyl metabolites. Application to bio-analysis.* In: Pinedo, J.M., ed., *Clinical Pharmacology of Antineoplastic Drugs,* Elsevier/North-Holland Biomedical Press, pp. 193–207

El Dareer, S.M., White, V.M., Chen, F.P., Mellet, L.B. & Hill, D.L. (1977) Distribution and metabolism of vincristine in mice, rats, dogs and monkeys. *Cancer Treatment Rep., 61(7),* 1269–1277

Ellaithy, M.M., El-Tarras, M.F., Tadros, N.B. & Amer, M.M. (1982) Analytical study of methotrexate. *Anal. Lett., 15(B11),* 981–988

Fell, A.F., Plag, S.M. & Neil, J.M. (1979) Stability-indicating assay for azathioprine and 6-mercaptopurine by reversed-phase high performance liquid chromatography. *J. Chromatogr., 186,* 691–704

Feyns, L.V., Thakker, K.D., Reif, V.D. & Grady, L.T. (1982) Purity profiles of pteroylglutamate reference substances by high performance liquid chromatography. *J. pharm. Sci., 71(11),* 1242–1246

Finkel, J.M., Knapp, K.T. & Mulligan, L.T. (1969) Fluorometric determination of serum levels and urinary excretion of daunomycin (NSC-82151) in mice and rats. *Cancer Chemother. Rep., 53(3)*, 159–164

Flora, K.P., Smith, S.L. & Craddock, J.C. (1979) Application of a simple high-performance liquid chromatographic method for the determination of melphalan in the presence of its hydrolysis products. *J. Chromatogr., 177*, 91–97

Friedman, O.M. (1967) Recent biologic and chemical studies of cyclophosphamide (NSC-26271). *Cancer Chemother. Rep., 51(6)*, 327–333

Friedman, O.M., Bien, S. & Chakrabarti, J.K. (1965) Studies on the hydrolysis of cyclophosphamide. I. Identification of N-(2-hydroxyethyl)-N'-(3-hydroxypropyl)ethylenediamine as the main product. *J. Am. chem. Soc., 87(21)*, 4978–4979

Gallelli, J.F. (1967) Stability studies of drugs used in intravenous solutions. *Am. J. Hosp. Pharm., 24*, 425–433

Gattavecchia, E., Tonelli, D., Ghini, S. & Breccia A. (1983) Thin layer chromatographic determination of ^{14}C-labelled and unlabelled cyclophosphamide. *Anal. Lett., 16 (B1)*, 57–67

Görög, S., Herényi, B. & Jovánovics, K. (1977) High-performance liquid chromatography of Catharanthus alkaloids. *J. Chromatogr., 139*, 203–206

Gray, P.J. & Phillips, D.R. (1981) Ultraviolet photoirradiation of daunomycin and DNA-daunomycin complexes. *Photochem. Photobiol., 33*, 297–303

Greene, R.F., Chatterji, D.C., Hiranaka, P.K. & Gallelli, J.F. (1979) Stability of cis-platin in aqueous solution. *Am. J. Hosp. Pharm., 36*, 38–43

Habs, M., Eisenbrand, G. & Schmael, D. (1979) Carcinogenic activity in Sprague-Dawley rats of 2-[3-(2-chloroethyl)-nitrosoureido]-D-glucopyranose(chlorozotocin). *Cancer Lett., 8*, 133–137

Handelsman, H., Goldsmith, M.A. & Slavik, M. (1974) *Isophosphamide NSC-109724, Clinical Brochure*, Bethesda, MD, National Cancer Institute, Division of Cancer Treatment

Haneke, A.C., Crawford, J. & Aszalos, A. (1981) Quantitation of daunorubicin, doxorubicin and their aglycones by ion-pair reversed phase chromatography. *J. pharm. Sci., 70(10)*, 1112–1115

Hansen, J., Kreilgárd, B., Nielsen, O. & Veje, J. (1983) Kinetics of degradation of methotrexate in aqueous solution. *Int. J. Pharmaceut., 16*, 141–152

Harrison, B.R. (1981) Developping guidelines for working with antineoplastic drugs. *Am. J. Hosp. Pharm., 38*, 1686–1693

Hassan, S.S.M. & Eldesouki, M.H. (1981) Spectrophotometric determination of phosphorous and arsenic in pharmaceutical organic compounds. *Mikro chim. Acta, II*, 261–267

Hayatsu, H., Oka, T., Wakata, A., Ohara, Y., Hayatsu, T., Kobayashi, H. & Arimoto, S. (1983) Adsorption of mutagens to cotton bearing covalently bound trisulfo-copper-phthalocyanine. *Mutat. Res., 119*, 233–238

Herr, R. R., Jahnke, H. K. & Argoudelis, A. D. (1967) The structure of streptozotocin. *J. Am. chem. Soc., 89(18)*, 4808–4809

Hincal, A.A., Long, D.F. & Repta, A.J. (1979) Cis-platin stability in aqueous parenteral vehicles. *J. Parenteral Drug Assoc., 33(3)*, 107–116

Hirose, T. & Tawa, R. (1983) An improved method for micro-fluorimetric determination of 6-mercaptopurine. *Anal. Lett., 16(B3)*, 209–218

Holdiness, K. R. & Morgan, L., Jr (1983) Electron capture-gas chromatographic analysis of ifosfamide in human plasma and urine. *J. Chromatogr., 275*, 432–435

Hóor, M. & Toth, Z. (1981) Direct volumetric determination of sulfates on the basis of sulfate ion using a lead nitrate volumetric solution and a dithizone indicator. *Gyogyszereszet, 25*, 454–457

Humphreys, A., Marty, J.J., Gooey, S.L. & Bourne, D.W.F. (1978) Stability of methotrexate in an intravenous fluid. *Aust. J. Hosp. Pharm., 8(2)*, 66–67

International Agency for Research on Cancer (1974) *IARC Monographs on the Evaluation of Carcinogenic Risk of Chemicals to Man*, Vol. 4, *Some Aromatic Amines, Hydrazines and Related Substances,* N-*Nitroso Compounds and Miscellaneous Alkylating Agents*, Lyon

International Agency for Research on Cancer (1975) *IARC Monographs on the Evaluation of Carcinogenic Risk of Chemicals to Man, Vol. 9, Some Aziridines,* N-, S- & O-*Mustards and Selenium*, Lyon

International Agency for Research on Cancer (1976) *IARC Monographs on the Evaluation of Carcinogenic Risk to Man, Vol. 10, Some Naturally Occurring Substances*, Lyon

International Agency for Research on Cancer (1978) *IARC Monographs on the Evaluation of the Carcinogenic Risk of Chemicals to Humans, Vol. 17, Some* N-*Nitroso Compounds*, Lyon

International Agency for Research on Cancer (1981) *IARC Monographs on the Evaluation of the Carcinogenic Risk of Chemicals to Humans, Vol. 26, Some Antineoplastic and Immunosuppressive Agents*, Lyon

International Agency for Research on Cancer (1982) *IARC Monographs on the Evaluation of the Carcinogenic Risk of Chemicals to Humans,* Supplement No. 4, *Chemicals, Industrial Processes and Industries Associated with Cancer in Humans IARC Monographs 1–29*, Lyon

Issaq, H.J., Barr, E.W., Wei, T., Meyers, C. & Aszalos, A. (1977) Thin layer chromatographic classification of antibiotics exhibiting antitumour properties. *J. Chromatogr., 133*, 291–301

Jackson, C., Jr & Reynolds, P.J. (1972) Gas chromatographic determination of cyclophosphamide residues in sheep tissues. *J. Agric. Food Chem., 20(5)*, 972–974

Jarman, M. (1973) Formation of 4-ketocyclophosphamide by the oxidation of cyclophosphamide with $KMnO_4$. *Experientia, 29(7)*, 812–814

Jensen, E.M., La Polla, R.J., Kirby, P.E. & Haworth, S.R. (1977) *In vitro* studies of chemical mutagens and carcinogens. I. Stability studies in cell culture medium. *J. natl Cancer Inst., 59(3),* 941–944

Johnston, T.P., McCaleb, G.S., Anderson, T. & Montgomery, J.A. (1975) Synthesis of chlorozotocin, the 2-chloroethylanalog of the anticancer antibiotic streptozotocin. *J. med. Chem., 18(1),* 104–106

Johnston, T.P., McCaleb, G.S., Anderson, T. & Murinson, D.S. (1979) L-Chlorozotocin. *J. med. Chem., 22(5),* 597–599

Jones, R.B., Frank, R. & Mass, T. (1983) Safe handling of chemotherapeutic agents: A report from the Mount Sinai Medical Center. *CA, 33,* 258–263

Jonkers, R.E., Oosterhuis, B., Ten Berge, R.J.M. & Van Boxtel, C.J. (1982) Analysis of 6-mercaptopurine in human plasma with high performance liquid chromatographic method including post column derivatization and fluorimetric detection. *J. Chromatogr., 233,* 249–255

Jovanovics, K., Szász, K., Fekete, G., Bittner, E., Dezséri, E. & Eles, J. (1975) *Chromic acid oxidation of vinblastine sulfate to form vincristine,* United States Patent No. 3,899,493

Karlsen, J., Thønnesen, H.H., Olsen, T.R., Sollien, A.H. & Skobba, T.J. (1983) Stability of cytotoxic intravenous solutions subjected to freeze-thaw treatment. *Nord. pharm. Acta, 45,* 61–67

Kauffman, G.B. & Cowan, D.O. (1963) *Cis- and trans-dichlorodiamine-platinum* (II). In: Kleinberg, J., ed., *Inorganic Synthesis,* Vol. 7, New York, McGraw-Hill, pp. 239–245

Keller, J.H. & Ensminger, W.D. (1982) Stability of chemotherapeutic agents in a totally inplanted drug delivery system. *Am. J. Hosp. Pharm., 39,* 3121–3123

Kensler, T.T., Behme, R.J. & Brooke, D. (1979) High performance liquid chromatographic analysis of cyclophosphamide. *J. pharm. Sci., 68(2),* 172–174

Knowles, R.S. & Virden, J.E. (1980) Handling the injectable antineoplastic agents. *Br. med. J., 281,* 589–591

Krull, I.S., Strauss, J., Hochberg, F. & Zervas, N.T. (1981) An improved trace analysis for *N*-nitrosoureas from biological media. *J. Anal. Toxicol., 5,* 42–46

Krull, I.S., Ding, X.D., Braverman, S., Selavka, C., Hochberg, F. & Sternson, L.A. (1983) Trace analysis for cis-platinum anti-cancer drugs via LCEC. *J. chromatogr. Sci., 21,* 166–173

Laskar, P.A. & Ayres, J.W. (1977a) Degradation of carmustine in aqueous media. *J. pharm. Sci., 66(8),* 1073–1076

Laskar, P.A. & Ayres, J.W. (1977b) Degradation of carmustine in mixed solvent and non aqueous media. *J. pharm. Sci., 66(8),* 1076–1078

Levy, C.C. & Goldman, P. (1967) The enzymatic hydrolysis of methotrexate and folic acid. *J. biol. Chem., 242(12),* 2933–2938

Loo, T. L. & Dion, R. L. (1965) Colorimetric method for the determination of 1,3-bis-(2-chloroethyl)-1-nitrosourea. *J. pharm. Sci., 54,* 809–810

Loo, T. L., Dion, R. L., Dixon, R. L. & Rall, D. P. (1966) The antitumor agent, 1,3-bis(2-chloroethyl)-1-nitrosourea. *J. pharm. Sci., 55(5),* 492–497

Lown, J. W. & Chauhan, S. M. S. (1981a) Synthesis of specifically [15]N- and ^{13}C-labelled antitumor (2-haloethyl)nitrosoureas. The study of their conformations in solution by nitrogen-15 and carbon-13 nuclear magnetic resonance and evidence for the stereoelectronic control in their aqueous decomposition. *J. org. Chem., 46,* 5309–5321

Lown, J. W. & Chauhan, S. M. S. (1981b) Mechanism of action of (2-haloethyl)nitrosoureas on DNA. Isolation and reaction of postulated 2-(alkylimino)-3-nitrosooxazolidine intermediates in the decomposition of 1,3-bis(2-chloroethyl)-, 1-(2-chloroethyl)-3-cyclohexyl-, and 1-(2-chloroethyl)-3-(4-*trans*-methylcyclohexyl)-1-nitrosourea. *J. med. Chem., 24,* 270–279

Lown, J. W. & Chauhan, S. M. S. (1982) Discrimination between alternative pathways of aqueous decomposition of antitumor (2-chloroethyl) nitroureas using specific [18]O labelling. *J. org. Chem., 47,* 851–856

Lown, J. W., McLaughlin, L. W. & Plambeck, J. A. (1979) Mechanism of action of 2-haloethylnitrosoureas on deoxyribonucleic acid. *Biochem. Pharmacol., 28,* 2115–2121

Ludeman, S. M., Zon, G. & Egan, W. (1979) Synthesis and antitumor activity of cyclophosphamide analogues. 2. Preparation, hydrolytic studies and anticancer screening of 5-bromocyclophosphamide, 3,5-dehydrocyclophosphamide, and related systems. *J. med. Chem., 22(2),* 151–158

Mariani, E. P., Southard, B. J., Woolever, J. T., Erlich, R. H. & Granatek, A. P. (1980) *Physical compatibility and chemical stability of cis-platin in various diluents and in large-volume parenteral solutions.* In: Prestayko, A. W., Crooke, S. T. & Carter, S. K., eds, *Cis-platin,* New York, Academic Press, pp. 305–316

Masaharu, H., Hirotane, K. & Masaya, B. (1967) Cyclophosphamide. I. Determination and degradation kinetics in aqueous media. *Shionogi Kenkgusho Nempo, 17,* 107–113

May, H. E., Boose, R. & Reed, D. J. (1975) Microsomal monooxygenation of the carcinostatic 1-(2-chloroethyl)-1-nitrosourea. Synthesis and identification of cis and trans monohydroxylated products. *Biochemistry, 14(21),* 4723–4730

May, P. M., Williams, G. K. & Williams, D. R. (1980) Solution chemistry studies of adriamycin-iron complexes present *in vivo. Eur. J. Cancer, 16,* 1275–1276

McKinley, W. A. (1981) Application of the photoconductivity detector to the liquid chromatographic analysis of pharmaceuticals in biological fluids. *J. anal. Toxicol., 5,* 209–215

Montgomery, J. A., James, R., McCaleb, G. S. & Johnston, T. P. (1967) The modes of decomposition of 1,3-bis(2-chloroethyl)-1-nitrosourea and related compounds. *J. med. Chem., 10,* 668–674

Montgomery, J.A., James, R., McCaleb, G.S., Kirk, M.C. & Johnston, T.P. (1975) Decomposition of *N*-(2-chloroethyl)-*N*-nitrosoureas in aqueous media. *J. med., Chem., 18(6),* 568–771

Morimoto, K., Yamaha, T., Nakadate, M. & Suzuki, I. (1978) Chemical stability, alkylating activity and lipophilicity of 1,1'-ethylene-bis(1-nitrosourea) and related compounds. *Gann, 69,* 139–142

Nakamura, K.I., Asami, M., Orita, S. & Kawada, K. (1979) Chromatographic studies on chemical degradation of carcinostatic nitrosoureas. *J. Chromatogr., 168,* 221–226

Narang, P.K., Yeager, R.L. & Chatterji, D.C. (1982) Quantitation of 6-mercaptopurine in biological fluids using high-performance liquid chromatography: A selective and novel procedure. *J. Chromatogr., 230,* 373–380

National Cancer Institute (1980) Experimental evaluation of antitumor drugs in the USA and USSR and clinical correlations. *Natl Cancer Inst Monogr.,* 55

National Cancer Institute (1983) *NCI Investigational Drugs, Pharmaceutical Data (NIH Publication No. 83–2141)*, Washington DC, Department of Health and Human Services, Public Health Service, National Institutes of Health

National Institutes of Health (1982) *Recommendations for the Safe Handling of Parenteral Antineoplastic Drugs,* Washington DC, Division of Safety, Public Health Service, Department of Health and Human Services

National Study Commission on Cytotoxic Exposure (1984) *Recommendations for Handling of Cytotoxic Agents (III),* Washington DC, US Government Printing Office

Norpoth, K., Knippschild, J., Witting, U. & Raven, H.M. (1972) Oxidation of cyclophosphamide by means of $KMnO_4$. *Experientia, 28(5),* 536–537

Pallante, S.L., Fenselau, C., Mennel, R.G., Brundrett, R.B., Appler, M., Rosenheim, N.B. & Colvin, M. (1980) Quantitation by gas chromatography-chemical ionization-mass spectrometry of phenylalanine mustard in bile plasma. *Cancer Res., 40,* 2268–2272

Panas, J.M., Etcheverry, M.F., Yzerman, J.M. & Ledouble, G. (1979) Dosage densitométrique d'impuretés alcaloïdiques dans le sulfate de vincristine. *Ann. Pharm. fr., 37(12),* 49–54

Panasci, L.C., Green, D., Nagourney, R., Fox, P. & Schein, P.S. (1977) A structure-activity analysis of chemical and biological parameters of chloroethylnitrosoureas in mice. *Cancer Res., 37,* 2615–2618

Pantarotto, C., Bossi, A., Belvedere, G., Martini, A., Donelli, M.G. & Frigerio, A. (1974) Quantitative GLC determination of cyclophosphamide and isophosphamide in biological specimens. *J. pharm. Sci., 63,* 1554–1558

Piall, E., Aherne, G.W. & Marks, V. (1982) Evaluation of commercially available radioimmunoassay kit for the measurement of doxorubicin in plasma. *Clin. Chem., 28(1),* 119–121

Pierce, R.N. & Jatlow, P.I. (1979) Measurement of adriamycin (doxorubicin) and its metabolites in human plasma using reversed-phase high performance liquid chromatography and fluorescence detection. *J. Chromatogr., 164,* 471–478

Priesner, D., Sternson, L.A. & Repta, A.J. (1981) Analysis of total platinum in tissue samples by flameless atomic absorption spectrophotometry. Elimination of the need for sample digestion. *Anal. Lett., 14,* 1255–1268

Przybylski, M., Preiss, J., Dennebaum, R. & Fischer, J. (1982) Identification and quantitation of methotrexate and methotrexate metabolites by high-pressure liquid chromatography and field desorption mass spectrometry. *Biochem. Mass Spectrom. 9(1),* 22–32

Reed, D.J., May, H.E., Boose, R.B., Gregory, K.M. & Beilstein, M.A. (1975) 2-Chloroethanol formation as evidence for a chloroethyl alkylating intermediate during chemical degradation of 1-(2-chloroethyl)-3-cyclohexyl-1-nitrosourea and 1-(2-chloroethyl)-3-(trans-4-methylcyclohexyl)-1-nitrosourea. *Cancer Res., 35,* 568–576

Repta, A.J., Long, D.F. & Hincal, A.A. (1979) Cis-dichlorodiamine-platinum (II) stability in aqueous vehicles. 'An alternate view'. *Cancer Treatment Rep., 63(2),* 229–230

Riley, C.M., Sternson, L.A. & Repta, A.J. (1981) High performance liquid chromatography of cis-dichlorodiammineplatinum (II) using chemically-bonded and solvent-generated ion exchangers. *J. Chromatogr., 217,* 405–420

Riley, C.M., Sternson, L.A., Repta, A.J. & Siegler, R.W. (1982) High performance liquid chromatography of platin complexes on solvent generated anion exchangers. III. Application to the analysis of cis-platin in urine using automated column switching. *J. Chromatogr., 229,* 373–386

Riley, C.M., Sternson, L.A. & Repta, A.J. (1983) High performance liquid chromatography of cis-platin. *J. pharm. Sci., 72(4),* 351–355

Robert, J. (1980) Extraction of anthracyclines from biological fluids for HPLC evaluation. *J. Liquid Chromatogr., 3(10),* 1561–1572

Rudas, B. (1972) Streptozotocin. *Arzneimittel-Forsch., 22,* 830–861

Rusling, J.F., Scheer, B.J. & Haque, I.V. (1984) Voltammetric oxidation of vinblastine and related compounds. *Anal. chim. Acta, 158,* 23–32

Schein, P.S., Heal, J., Green, D. & Woolley, P.V. (1978) Pharmacology of nitrosourea antitumor agents. *Fundam. Cancer Chemother. Antibiot. Chemother., 23,* 64–75

Scheufler, E. (1981) Improved enzymatic assay for methotrexate: shape of standard curve, stability of reagents, sensitivity. *Clin. chim. Acta, 111,* 113–116

Schwartz, H.S. (1973) Fluorometric assay for daunomycin and adriamycin in animal tissues. *Biochem. Med., 7(3),* 396–404

Sepaniak, M.J. & Yeung, E.S. (1980) Determination of adriamycin and daunorubicin in urine by high performance liquid chromatography with laser fluorometric detection. *J. Chromatogr., 190,* 377–383

Shinozawa, S. & Oda, T. (1981) Determination of adriamycin (doxorubicin) and related fluorescent compounds in rat lymph and gall by high performance liquid chromatography. *J. Chromatogr., 212,* 323–330

Smith, R.G. & Cheung, L.K. (1982) Determination of two nitrosourea antitumor agents by chemical ionization gas chromatography-mass spectrometry. *J. Chromatogr., 229,* 464–469

Smith, D.L. & Elving, P.J. (1962) Analytical utilization of polarographic and voltammetric behaviour of purines and pyrimidines. *Anal. Chem., 34,* 930–936

Smith, T.H., Fujiwara, A.N., Lee, W.W., Wu, H.Y. & Henry, D.W. (1977) Synthetic approaches to adriamycin. 2. Degradation of daunorubicin to a nonasymmetric tetracyclic ketone and refunctionalization of the ring to adriamycin. *J. org. Chem., 42(23),* 3653–3660

Smith, R.G., Blackstock, S.C., Cheung, L.K. & Loo, T.L. (1981) Analysis for nitrosourea antitumor agents by gas chromatography-mass spectrometry. *Anal. Chem., 53,* 1205–1208

Solimando, D.A., Jr (1983) Preparation of antineoplastic drugs: A review. *Am. J. IV Ther. Clin. Nutr., 10,* 16–27

Stolar, M.H., Power, L.A. & Viele, C.S. (1983) Recommendations for handling cytotoxic drugs in hospitals. *Am. J. Hosp. Pharm., 40,* 1163–1171

Struck, R.F., Thorpe, M.C., Coburn, W.C., Jr & Laster, W.R., Jr (1974) Cyclophosphamide. Complete inhibition of murine leukemia L 1210 *in vivo* by a Fenton oxidation product. *J. Am. chem. Soc., 96(1),* 313–315

Takamizawa, A., Matsumoto, S. & Iwata, T. (1974) 4-Hydroxycyclophosphamide anhydrodimer: revised structure of the Fenton oxidation product of cyclophosphamide. *Tetrahedron Lett., 6,* 517–524

Tavoloni, N., Guarino, A.M. & Berk, P.D. (1980) Photolytic degradation of adriamycin. *J. Pharm. Pharmacol., 32,* 860–862

Thomson, M. & Colvin, M. (1974) Chemical oxidation of cyclophosphamide and 4-methylcyclophosphamide. *Cancer Res., 34,* 981–985

Tong, G., Lee, W.W., Black, D.R. & Henry, D.W. (1976) Adriamycin analogs. Periodate oxidation of adriamycin. *J. med. Chem., 19(3),* 395–398

Tsutsumi, K., Otsuki, Y. & Kinoshita, T. (1982) Simultaneous determination of azathioprine and 6-mercaptopurine in serum by reversed-phase high performance liquid chromatography. *J. Chromatogr., 231,* 393–399

Vachek, J., Svátek, E. & Kakáč, B. (1982) Spektrofotometrické a polarografiké stanoveni lomustinu. *Cesk. Farm., 31(9),* 351–352

Van den Bosch, N., Driessen, O., Emonds, A., Van Oosterom, A.T., Timmermans, P.J.A., De Vos, D. & Slee, P.H.Th.J. (1981) Determination of plasma concentrations of underivatized cyclophosphamide by capillary gas chromatography. *Meth. Fund. exp. clin. Pharmacol., 3(6),* 377–384

Van der Steen, J., Timmer, E.C., Westra, J.G. & Benckhuysen, C. (1973) 4-Hydroperoxidation in the Fenton oxidation of the antitumor agent cyclophosphamide. *J. Am. chem. Soc., 95(22),* 7535–7536

Vigevani, A. & Williamson, M.J. (1980) *Doxorubicin.* In: Florey, K., ed. *Analytical Profiles of Drug Substances,* Vol. 9, New York, Academic Press, pp. 245–274

Völker, von G., Dräger, V., Peter, G. & Hohorst, H.J. (1974) Studien zum Spontanzer Fall von 4-Hydroxycyclophosphamid und 4-Hydroperoxycyclophosphamid mit Hilfe der Dünnschichtchromatographie. *Arzneimittel-Forsch., 24(8),* 1172–1176

Vrána, O., Kleinwächter, V. & Brabec, V. (1983) Determination of platinum in urine by differential pulse polarography. *Talanta, 30(4),* 288–290

Wade, A., ed. (1977) *Martindale, The Extra Pharmacopoeia,* 27th ed., London, The Pharmaceutical Press

Weast, R.C., ed. (1977) *Handbook of Chemistry and Physics,* 58th ed., Cleveland, OH, The Chemical Rubber Company

Weinkam, R.J. & Liu, T-Y.J. (1982) Quantitation of lipophilic chloronitrosourea cancer chemotherapeutic agents. *J. pharm. Sci., 71(2),* 153–157

Weinkam, R.J., Wen, J.H.C., Furst, D.E. & Levin, V.A. (1978) Analysis of 1,3-bis(2-chloroethyl)-1-nitrosourea by chemical ionisation mass spectrometry. *Clin. Chem., 24(1),* 45–49

White, F.R. (1963) Streptozotocin. *Cancer Chemother. Rep., 30,* 49–59

White, E.R. & Zarembo, J.E. (1981) Reverse phase high speed liquid chromatography of antibiotics. III. Use of ultra high performance columns and ion pairing techniques. *J. Antibiot., 34(7),* 836–844

Whiting, B., Miller, S.H.K. & Caddy, B. (1978) A procedure for monitoring cyclophosphamide and isophosphamide in biological samples. *J. clin. Pharmacol., 6,* 373–376

Windholz, M., ed. (1983) *The Merck Index,* 10th ed., Rahway, NJ, Merck & Co.

Woodhouse, K.W. & Henderson, D.B. (1982) High pressure liquid chromatographic method for the determination of melphalan in plasma. *Br. J. clin. Pharmacol., 13(4),* 605 P

Yoshida, K. & Yano, K. (1983) Kinetic study of decomposition of *N*-(2-haloethyl)-cyclohexyl-*N*-nitrosoureas. Effect of haloethyl group on the preference in decomposition pathways. *Bull. chem. Soc. Jpn., 56,* 1557–1558

Zimmerman, P.F., Larsen, R.K., Barkley, W.E. & Gallelli, J.F. (1981) Recommendations for the safe handling of injectable antineoplastic drug products. *Am. J. Hosp. Pharm., 38,* 1693–1695

Zon, G., Ludeman, S.M. & Egan, W. (1977) High resolution nuclear magnetic resonance investigations of the chemical stability of cyclophosphamide and related phosphoramidic compounds. *J. Am. chem. Soc., 99(17),* 5785–5795

ERRATUM

Laboratory Decontamination and Destruction of Carcinogens in Laboratory Wastes: Some Hydrazines (IARC Scientific Publications No. 54)

p. 49   Section 1, after paragraph 3   *Insert:* Residues of degradation of hydrazines by this method have been tested for mutagenic activity using *Salmonella typhimurium* strains TA1530, TA1535 and TA100 and in addition TA98 for residues from procarbazine. With sodium hypochlorite treatment, only MMH gave non-mutagenic residues, while with calcium hypochlorite non-mutagenic residues were obtained from MMH, hydrazine and procarbazine. All other residues exerted some mutagenic activity.

PUBLICATIONS OF THE INTERNATIONAL AGENCY FOR RESEARCH ON CANCER

SCIENTIFIC PUBLICATIONS SERIES

(Available from Oxford University Press)

No. 1 LIVER CANCER (1971)
176 pages; £10-

No. 2 ONCOGENESIS AND HERPES
VIRUSES (1972)
Edited by P.M. Biggs, G. de Thé &
L.N. Payne
515 pages; £30.-

No. 3 N-NITROSO COMPOUNDS -
ANALYSIS AND FORMATION (1972)
Edited by P. Bogovski, R. Preussmann
& E.A. Walker
140 pages; £8.50

No. 4 TRANSPLACENTAL
CARCINOGENESIS (1973)
Edited by L. Tomatis & U. Mohr,
181 pages; £11.95

No. 5 PATHOLOGY OF TUMOURS IN
LABORATORY ANIMALS. VOLUME 1.
TUMOURS OF THE RAT. PART 1 (1973)
Editor-in-Chief V.S. Turusov
214 pages; £17.50

No. 6 PATHOLOGY OF TUMOURS IN
LABORATORY ANIMALS. VOLUME 1.
TUMOURS OF THE RAT. PART 2 (1976)
Editor-in-Chief V.S. Turusov
319 pages; £17.50

No. 7 HOST ENVIRONMENT INTER-
ACTIONS IN THE ETIOLOGY OF
CANCER IN MAN (1973)
Edited by R. Doll & I. Vodopija,
464 pages; £30.-

No. 8 BIOLOGICAL EFFECTS OF
ASBESTOS (1973)
Edited by P. Bogovski, J.C. Gilson,
V. Timbrell & J.C. Wagner,
346 pages; £25.-

No. 9 N-NITROSO COMPOUNDS IN
THE ENVIRONMENT (1974)
Edited by P. Bogovski & E.A. Walker
243 pages; £15.-

No. 10 CHEMICAL CARCINOGENESIS
ESSAYS (1974)
Edited by R. Montesano & L. Tomatis,
230 pages; £15.-

No. 11 ONCOGENESIS AND HERPES-
VIRUSES II (1975)
Edited by G. de-Thé, M.A. Epstein
& H. zur Hausen
Part 1, 511 pages; £30.-
Part 2, 403 pages; £30.-

No. 12 SCREENING TESTS IN
CHEMICAL CARCINOGENESIS (1976)
Edited by R. Montesano, H. Bartsch &
L. Tomatis
666 pages; £30.-

No. 13 ENVIRONMENTAL POLLUTION
AND CARCINOGENIC RISKS (1976)
Edited by C. Rosenfeld & W. Davis
454 pages; £17.50

No. 14 ENVIRONMENTAL N-NITROSO
COMPOUNDS - ANALYSIS AND
FORMATION (1976)
Edited by E.A. Walker, P. Bogovski &
L. Griciute
512 pages; £35.-

No. 15 CANCER INCIDENCE IN FIVE
CONTINENTS. VOL. III (1976)
Edited by J. Waterhouse, C.S. Muir,
P. Correa & J. Powell
584 pages; £35.-

No. 16 AIR POLLUTION AND CANCER
IN MAN (1977)
Edited by U. Mohr, D. Schmahl &
L. Tomatis
331 pages; £30.-

No. 17 DIRECTORY OF ON-GOING
RESEARCH IN CANCER EPI-
DEMIOLOGY 1977 (1977)
Edited by C.S. Muir & G. Wagner,
599 pages; out of print

No. 18 ENVIRONMENTAL CARCINO-
GENS - SELECTED METHODS OF
ANALYSIS
Editor-in-Chief H. Egan
Vol. 1 - ANALYSIS OF VOLATILE
NITROSAMINES IN FOOD (1978)
Edited by R. Preussmann,
M. Castegnaro, E.A. Walker
& A.E. Wassermann
212 pages; £30.-

SCIENTIFIC PUBLICATIONS SERIES

No. 19 ENVIRONMENTAL ASPECTS
OF N-NITROSO COMPOUNDS (1978)
Edited by E.A. Walker, M. Castegnaro,
L. Griciute & R.E. Lyle
566 pages; £35.-

No. 20 NASOPHARYNGEAL
CARCINOMA: ETIOLOGY AND
CONTROL (1978)
Edited by G. de-Thé & Y. Ito,
610 pages; £35.-

No. 21 CANCER REGISTRATION
AND ITS TECHNIQUES (1978)
Edited by R. MacLennan, C.S. Muir,
R. Steinitz & A. Winkler
235 pages;
£11.95

No. 22 ENVIRONMENTAL CARCINO-
GENS - SELECTED METHODS OF
ANALYSIS
Editor-in-Chief H. Egan
Vol. 2 - METHODS FOR THE MEASURE-
MENT OF VINYL CHLORIDE IN
POLY(VINYL CHLORIDE), AIR, WATER
AND FOODSTUFFS (1978)
Edited by D.C.M. Squirrell & W. Thain,
142 pages; £35.-

No. 23 PATHOLOGY OF TUMOURS IN
LABORATORY ANIMALS. VOLUME II.
TUMOURS OF THE MOUSE (1979)
Editor-in-Chief V.S. Turusov
669 pages; £35.-

No. 24 ONCOGENESIS AND HERPES-
VIRUSES III (1978)
Edited by G. de-Thé, W. Henle & F. Rapp
Part 1, 580 pages; £20.-
Part 2, 522 pages; £20.-

No. 25 CARCINOGENIC RISKS -
STRATEGIES FOR INTERVENTION
(1979)
Edited by W. Davis & C. Rosenfeld,
283 pages; £20.-

No. 26 DIRECTORY OF ON-GOING
RESEARCH IN CANCER EPI-
DEMIOLOGY 1978 (1978)
Edited by C.S. Muir & G. Wagner,
550 pages; out of print

No. 27 MOLECULAR AND CELLULAR
ASPECTS OF CARCINOGEN
SCREENING TESTS (1980)
Edited by R. Montesano, H. Bartsch &
L. Tomatis
371 pages; £20.-

No. 28 DIRECTORY OF ON-GOING
RESEARCH IN CANCER EPI-
DEMIOLOGY 1979 (1979)
Edited by C.S. Muir & G. Wagner,
672 pages; out of print

No. 29 ENVIRONMENTAL CARCINO-
GENS - SELECTED METHODS OF
ANALYSIS
Editor-in-Chief H. Egan
Vol. 3 - ANALYSIS OF POLYCYCLIC
AROMATIC HYDROCARBONS IN
ENVIRONMENTAL SAMPLES (1979)
Edited by M. Castegnaro, P. Bogovski,
H. Kunte & E.A. Walker
240 pages; £17.50

No. 30 BIOLOGICAL EFFECTS OF
MINERAL FIBRES (1980)
Editor-in-Chief J.C. Wagner
Volume 1, 494 pages; £25.-
Volume 2, 513 pages; £25.-

No. 31 N-NITROSO COMPOUNDS:
ANALYSIS, FORMATION AND
OCCURRENCE (1980)
Edited by E.A. Walker, M. Castegnaro,
L. Griciute & M. Börzsönyi
841 pages; £30.-

No. 32 STATISTICAL METHODS IN
CANCER RESEARCH
Vol. 1. THE ANALYSIS OF CASE-
CONTROL STUDIES (1980)
By N.E. Breslow & N.E. Day
338 pages; £17.50

No. 33 HANDLING CHEMICAL
CARCINOGENS IN THE LABORATORY
- PROBLEMS OF SAFETY (1979)
Edited by R. Montesano, H. Bartsch,
E. Boyland, G. Della Porta, L. Fishbein,
R.A. Griesemer, A.B. Swan & L. Tomatis,
32 pages; £3.95

No. 34 PATHOLOGY OF TUMOURS
IN LABORATORY ANIMALS. VOLUME
III. TUMOURS OF THE HAMSTER
(1982)
Editor-in-Chief V.S. Turusov,
461 pages; £30.-

No. 35 DIRECTORY OF ON-GOING
RESEARCH IN CANCER EPI-
DEMIOLOGY 1980 (1980)
Edited by C.S. Muir & G. Wagner,
660 pages; out of print

SCIENTIFIC PUBLICATIONS SERIES

No. 36 CANCER MORTALITY BY
OCCUPATION AND SOCIAL CLASS
1851-1971 (1982)
By W.P.D. Logan
253 pages £20.-

No. 37 LABORATORY DECONTAMI-
NATION AND DESTRUCTION OF
AFLATOXINS B_1, B_2, G_1, G_2 IN
LABORATORY WASTES (1980)
Edited by M. Castegnaro, D.C. Hunt,
E.B. Sansone, P.L. Schuller,
M.G. Siriwardana, G.M. Telling,
H.P. Van Egmond & E.A. Walker,
59 pages; £5.95

No. 38 DIRECTORY OF ON-GOING
RESEARCH IN CANCER EPI-
DEMIOLOGY 1981 (1981)
Edited by C.S. Muir & G. Wagner,
696 pages; out of print

No. 39 HOST FACTORS IN HUMAN
CARCINOGENESIS (1982)
Edited by H. Bartsch & B. Armstrong
583 pages; £35.-

No. 40 ENVIRONMENTAL CAR-
CINOGENS. SELECTED METHODS
OF ANALYSIS
Editor-in-Chief H. Egan
Vol. 4. SOME AROMATIC AMINES AND
AZO DYES IN THE GENERAL AND
INDUSTRIAL ENVIRONMENT (1981)
Edited by L. Fishbein, M. Castegnaro,
I.K. O'Neill & H. Bartsch
347 pages; £20.-

No. 41 N-NITROSO COMPOUNDS:
OCCURRENCE AND BIOLOGICAL
EFFECTS (1982)
Edited by H. Bartsch, I.K. O'Neill,
M. Castegnaro & M. Okada,
755 pages; £35.-

No. 42 CANCER INCIDENCE IN FIVE
CONTINENTS. VOLUME IV (1982)
Edited by J. Waterhouse, C. Muir,
K. Shanmugaratnam & J. Powell,
811 pages; £35.-

No. 43 LABORATORY DECONTAMI-
NATION AND DESTRUCTION OF
CARCINOGENS IN LABORATORY
WASTES: SOME N-NITROSAMINES
(1982) Edited by M. Castegnaro,
G. Eisenbrand, G. Ellen, L. Keefer,
D. Klein, E.B. Sansone, D. Spincer,
G. Telling & K. Webb
73 pages; £6.50

No. 44 ENVIRONMENTAL CAR-
CINOGENS. SELECTED METHODS
OF ANALYSIS
Editor-in-Chief H. Egan
Vol. 5. SOME MYCOTOXINS (1983)
Edited by L. Stoloff, M. Castegnaro,
P. Scott, I.K. O'Neill & H. Bartsch,
455 pages; £20.-

No. 45 ENVIRONMENTAL CAR-
CINOGENS. SELECTED METHODS
OF ANALYSIS
Editor-in-Chief H. Egan
Vol. 6: N-NITROSO COMPOUNDS
(1983)
Edited by R. Preussmann, I.K. O'Neill,
G. Eisenbrand, B. Spiegelhalder &
H. Bartsch
508 pages; £20.-

No. 46 DIRECTORY OF ON-GOING
RESEARCH IN CANCER EPI-
DEMIOLOGY 1982 (1982)
Edited by C.S. Muir & G. Wagner,
722 pages; out of print

No. 47 CANCER INCIDENCE IN
SINGAPORE (1982)
Edited by K. Shanmugaratnam, H.P. Lee
& N.E. Day
174 pages; £10.-

No. 48 CANCER INCIDENCE IN
THE USSR Second Revised
Edition (1983)
Edited by N.P. Napalkov,
G.F. Tserkovny, V.M. Merabishvili,
D.M. Parkin, M. Smans & C.S. Muir,
75 pages; £10.-

No. 49 LABORATORY DECONTAMI
NATION AND DESTRUCTION OF
CARCINOGENS IN LABORATORY
WASTES: SOME POLYCYCLIC
AROMATIC HYDROCARBONS (1983)
Edited by M. Castegnaro, G. Grimmer,
O. Hutzinger, W. Karcher, H. Kunte,
M. Lafontaine, E.B. Sansone, G. Telling
& S.P. Tucker
81 pages; £7.95

No. 50 DIRECTORY OF ON-GOING
RESEARCH IN CANCER
EPIDEMIOLOGY 1983 (1983)
Edited by C.S. Muir & G. Wagner,
740 pages; out of print

SCIENTIFIC PUBLICATIONS SERIES

No. 51 MODULATORS OF
EXPERIMENTAL CARCINO-
GENESIS (1983)
Edited by V. Turusov & R. Montesano
307 pages; £25.-

No. 52 SECOND CANCER IN
RELATION TO RADIATION
TREATMENT FOR CERVICAL
CANCER: RESULTS OF A CANCER
REGISTRY COLLABORATION (1984)
Edited by N.E. Day & J.C. Boice, Jr,
207 pages; £17.50

No. 53 NICKEL IN THE HUMAN
ENVIRONMENT (1984)
Editor-in-Chief, F.W. Sunderman, Jr,
529 pages; £30.-

No. 54 LABORATORY
DECONTAMINATION AND
DESTRUCTION OF CARCINO-
GENS IN LABORATORY WASTES:
SOME HYDRAZINES (1983)
Edited by M. Castegnaro, G. Ellen,
M. Lafontaine, H.C. van der Plas,
E.B. Sansone & S.P. Tucker,
87 pages; £6.95

No. 55 LABORATORY
DECONTAMINATION AND
DESTRUCTION OF CARCINOGENS
IN LABORATORY WASTES: SOME
N-NITROSAMIDES (1984)
Edited by M. Castegnaro,
M. Benard, L.W. van Broekhoven,
D. Fine, R. Massey, E.B. Sansone,
P.L.R. Smith, B. Spiegelhalder,
A. Stacchini, G. Telling & J.J. Vallon,
65 pages; £6.95

No. 56 MODELS, MECHANISMS AND
ETIOLOGY OF TUMOUR PROMOTION
(1984)
Edited by M. Börszönyi, N.E. Day,
K. Lapis & H. Yamasaki
532 pages, £30.-

No. 57 N-NITROSO COMPOUNDS:
OCCURRENCE, BIOLOGICAL EFFECTS
AND RELEVANCE TO HUMAN
CANCER (1984)
Edited by I.K. O'Neill, R.C. von Borstel,
C.T. Miller, J. Long & H. Bartsch,
1013 pages, £75.-

No. 58 AGE-RELATED FACTORS
IN CARCINOGENESIS (1985)
Edited by A. Likhachev, V. Anisimov
& R. Montesano
288 pages; £20.-

No. 59 MONITORING HUMAN
EXPOSURE TO CARCINOGENIC AND
MUTAGENIC AGENTS (1984)
Edited by A. Berlin, M. Draper,
K. Hemminki & H. Vainio
457 pages; £25.-

No. 60 BURKITT'S LYMPHOMA: A
HUMAN CANCER MODEL (1985)
Edited by G. Lenoir, G. O'Conor
& C.L.M. Olweny
484 pages; £25.-

No. 61 LABORATORY DECONTAMI-
NATION AND DESTRUCTION OF
CARCINOGENS IN LABORATORY
WASTES: SOME HALOETHERS (1984)
Edited by M. Castegnaro,
M. Alvarez, M. Iovu, E.B. Sansone,
G.M. Telling & D.T. Williams
55 pages, £5.95

No. 62 DIRECTORY OF ON-GOING
RESEARCH IN CANCER EPI-
DEMIOLOGY 1984 (1984)
Edited by C.S. Muir & G.Wagner
728 pages; £18.-

No. 63 VIRUS-ASSOCIATED CANCERS
IN AFRICA (1984)
Edited by A.O. Williams, G.T. O'Conor,
G.B. de-Thé & C.A. Johnson,
773 pages; £20.-

No. 64 LABORATORY DECONTAMI-
NATION AND DESTRUCTION OF
CARCINOGENS IN LABORATORY
WASTES: SOME AROMATIC AMINES
AND 4-NITROBIPHENYL (1985)
Edited by M. Castegnaro, J. Barek,
J. Dennis, G. Ellen, M. Klibanov,
M. Lafontaine, R. Mitchum,
P. Van Roosmalen, E.B. Sansone,
L.A. Sternson & M. Vahl
85 pages; £5.95

No. 65 INTERPRETATION OF
NEGATIVE EPIDEMIOLOGICAL
EVIDENCE FOR CARCINOGENICITY
Edited by N.J. Wald & R. Doll
232 pages; £20.-

No. 66 THE ROLE OF THE REGISTRY
IN CANCER CONTROL
Edited by D.M. Parkin, G. Wagner
& C.S. Muir (in press)

No. 67 TRANSFORMATION ASSAY OF
ESTABLISHED CELL LINES:
MECHANISMS AND APPLICATIONS
Edited by T. Kakunaga & H. Yamasaki
(in press)

SCIENTIFIC PUBLICATIONS SERIES

No. 68 ENVIRONMENTAL
CARCINOGENS — SELECTED
METHODS OF ANALYSIS.
VOL. 7: SOME VOLATILE
HALOGENATED ALKANES AND
ALKENES
Edited by L. Fishbein & I.K. O'Neill
479 pages; £20.-

No. 69 DIRECTORY OF ON-GOING
RESEARCH IN CANCER
EPIDEMIOLOGY 1985 (1985)
Edited by C.S. Muir & G. Wagner
756 pages; £22.-

No. 70 THE ROLE OF CYCLIC NUCLEIC
ACID ADDUCTS IN CARCINOGENESIS
AND MUTAGENESIS
Edited by B. Singer & H. Bartsch
(in press)

No. 71 ENVIRONMENTAL CARCINOGENS.
SELECTED METHODS OF ANALYSIS
VOL. 8:. SOME METALS: As, Be, Cd,
Cr, Ni, Pb, Se, Zn
Edited by I.K. O'Neill, P. Schuller
& L. Fishbein (in press)

No. 72 ATLAS OF CANCER IN
SCOTLAND 1975-1980: INCIDENCE AND
EPIDEMIOLOGICAL PERSPECTIVE (1985)
Edited by I. Kemp, P. Boyle, M. Smans
& C. Muir
282 pages; £30.-

No. 73 LABORATORY DECONTAMI-
NATION AND DESTRUCTION OF
CARCINOGENS IN LABORATORY
WASTES: SOME ANTINEOPLASTIC
AGENTS
Edited by M. Castegnaro, J. Adams,
M. Armour, J. Barek, J. Benvenuto,
C. Confalonieri, U. Goff, S. Ludeman,
D. Reed, E.B. Sansone & G. Telling
(1985)

NON-SERIAL PUBLICATIONS

(Available from IARC)

ALCOOL ET CANCER (1978)
By A.J. Tuyns (in French only)
42 pages; Fr.fr. 35.-; Sw.fr. 14.-

CANCER MORBIDITY AND CAUSES OF
DEATH AMONG DANISH BREWERY
WORKERS (1980)
By O.M. Jensen
145 pages; US$ 25.00; Sw.fr. 45.-

IARC MONOGRAPHS ON THE EVALUATION OF THE
CARCINOGENIC RISK OF CHEMICALS TO HUMANS
(English editions only)

(Available from WHO Sales Agents)

Volume 1
Some inorganic substances, chlorinated hydrocarbons, aromatic amines, N-nitroso compounds, and natural products (1972)
184 pp.; out of print

Volume 2
Some inorganic and organometallic compounds (1973)
181 pp.; out of print

Volume 3
Certain polycyclic aromatic hydrocarbons and heterocyclic compounds (1973)
271 pp.; out of print

Volume 4
Some aromatic amines, hydrazine and related substances, N-nitroso compounds and miscellaneous alkylating agents (1974)
286 pp.; US$7.20; Sw.fr. 18.-

Volume 5
Some organochlorine pesticides (1974)
241 pp.; out of print

Volume 6
Sex hormones (1974)
243 pp.; US$7.20; Sw.fr. 18.-

Volume 7
Some anti-thyroid and related substances, nitrofurans and industrial chemicals (1974)
326 pp.; US$12.80; Sw.fr. 32.-

Volume 8
Some aromatic azo compounds (1975)
357 pp.; US$14.40; Sw.fr. 36.-

Volume 9
Some aziridines, N-, S- and O-mustards and selenium (1975)
268 pp.; US$10.80; Sw.fr. 27.-

Volume 10
Some naturally occurring substances (1976)
353 pp.; US$15.00; Sw.fr. 38.-

Volume 11
Cadmium, nickel, some epoxides, miscellaneous industrial chemicals and general considerations on volatile anaesthetics (1976)
306 pp.; US$14.00; Sw.fr. 34.-

Volume 12
Some carbamates, thiocarbamates and carbazides (1976)
282 pp.; US$14.00; Sw.fr. 34.-

Volume 13
Some miscellaneous pharmaceutical substances (1977)
255 pp.; US$12.00; Sw.fr. 30.-

Volume 14
Asbestos (1977)
106 pp.; US$6.00; Sw.fr. 14.-

Volume 15
Some fumigants, the herbicides 2,4-D and 2,4,5-T, chlorinated dibenzodioxins and miscellaneous industrial chemicals (1977)
354 pp.; US$20.00; Sw.fr. 50.-

Volume 16
Some aromatic amines and related nitro compounds - hair dyes, colouring agents and miscellaneous industrial chemicals (1978)
400 pp.; US$20.00; Sw.fr. 50.-

Volume 17
Some N-nitroso compounds (1978)
365 pp.; US$25.00; Sw.fr. 50.-

Volume 18
Polychlorinated biphenyls and poly brominated biphenyls (1978)
140 pp.; US$13.00; Sw.fr. 20.-

Volume 19
Some monomers, plastics and synthetic elastomers, and acrolein (1979)
513 pp.; US$35.00; Sw.fr. 60.-

Volume 20
Some halogenated hydrocarbons (1979)
609 pp.; US$35.00; Sw.fr. 60.-

Volume 21
Sex hormones (II) (1979)
583 pp.; US$35.00; Sw.fr. 60.-

Volume 22
Some non-nutritive sweetening agents (1980)
208 pp.; US$15.00; Sw.fr. 25.-

IARC MONOGRAPHS SERIES

Volume 23
Some metals and metallic compounds (1980)
438 pp.; US$30.00; Sw.fr. 50.-

Volume 24
Some pharmaceutical drugs (1980)
337 pp.; US$25.00; Sw.fr. 40.-

Volume 25
Wood, leather and some associated industries (1981)
412 pp.; US$30.00; Sw.fr. 60.-

Volume 26
Some antineoplastic and immuno-suppressive agents (1981)
411 pp.; US$30.00; Sw.fr. 62.-

Volume 27
Some aromatic amines, anthraquinones and nitroso compounds, and inorganic fluorides used in drinking-water and dental preparations (1982)
341 pp.; US$25.00; Sw.fr. 40.-

Volume 28
The rubber industry (1982)
486 pp.; US$35.00; Sw.fr. 70.-

Volume 29
Some industrial chemicals and dyestuffs (1982)
416 pp.; US$30.00; Sw.fr. 60.-

Volume 30
Miscellaneous pesticides (1983)
424 pp; US$30.00; Sw.fr. 60.-

Volume 31
Some food additives, feed additives and naturally occurring substances (1983)
314 pp.; US$30.00; Sw.fr. 60.-

Volume 32
Polynuclear aromatic compounds, Part 1, Environmental and experimental data (1984)
477 pp.; US$30.00; Sw.fr. 60.-

Volume 33
Polynuclear aromatic compounds, Part 2, Carbon blacks, mineral oils and some nitroarene compounds (1984)
245 pp.; US$25.00; Sw.fr. 50.-

Volume 34
Polynuclear aromatic compounds, Part 3, Industrial exposures in aluminium production, coal gasification, coke production, and iron and steel founding (1984)
219 pages; US$20.00; Sw.fr. 48.-

Volume 35
Polynuclear aromatic compounds, Part 4, Bitumens, coal-tar and derived products, shale-oils and soots (1985)
271 pages; US$25.00; Sw.fr. 70.-

Volume 36
Allyl Compounds, aldehydes, epoxides and peroxides (1985)
369 pages; US$25.00; Sw.fr. 70.-

Volume 37
Tobacco habits other than smoking; betel-quid and areca-nut chewing; and some related nitrosamines (1985)
291 pages; US$25.00; Sw.fr. 70.-

Volume 38
Tobacco smoking (1985)
(in preparation)

Supplement No. 1
Chemicals and industrial processes associated with cancer in humans (IARC Monographs, Volumes 1 to 20) (1979)
71 pp.; out of print

Supplement No. 2
Long-term and short-term screening assays for carcinogens: a critical appraisal (1980)
426 pp.; US$25.00; Sw.fr. 40.-

Supplement No. 3
Cross index of synonyms and trade names in Volumes 1 to 26 (1982)
199 pp.; US$30.00; Sw.fr. 60.-

Supplement No. 4
Chemicals, industrial processes and industries associated with cancer in humans (IARC Monographs, Volumes 1 to 29) (1982)
292 pp.; US$30.00; Sw.fr. 60.-

INFORMATION BULLETINS ON THE
SURVEY OF CHEMICALS BEING
TESTED FOR CARCINOGENICITY

(Available from IARC)

No. 8 (1979)
Edited by M.-J. Ghess, H. Bartsch
& L. Tomatis
604 pp.; US$20.00; Sw.fr. 40.-

No. 9 (1981)
Edited by M.-J. Ghess, J.D. Wilbourn,
H. Bartsch & L. Tomatis
294 pp.; US$20.00; Sw.fr. 41.-

No. 10 (1982)
Edited by M.-J. Ghess, J.D. Wilbourn
H. Bartsch
326 pp.; US$20.00; Sw.fr. 42.-

No. 11 (1984)
Edited by M.-J. Ghess, J.D. Wilbourn,
H. Vainio & H. Bartsch
336 pp.; US$20.00; Sw.fr. 48.-